About the Author

Oscar Hofman, a phlegmatic choleric with a very strong Saturnian bent, was born just before the eclipse of February 1962, when there were almost too many planets in Aquarius. He studied chemistry and philosophy and worked as a journalist and a translator before he started his full-time astrological practice. He received his astrological schooling from John Frawley and as an all-round astrologer, he practises all the forms of traditional astrology: horary, electional, medical, natal and mundane. He lectures at conferences around the world, and has clients and students in many countries from Australia to Russia, from Japan to the US.

As an astrology teacher he runs a school which teaches three courses - in classical horary astrology, classical medical astrology, and classical natal/electional astrology - in four languages: Dutch, German, English and French. With George van Zanten he edits the Dutch magazine *Anima Astrologiae*. He writes columns for several magazines around the world.

He can be reached through: oshofman@xs4all.nl or info@pegasus-advies. com. Information about the astrology courses and the conference agenda can be found on his website: www.pegasus-advies.com.

CLASSICAL MEDICAL ASTROLOGY:

HEALING WITH THE ELEMENTS

Oscar Hofman

The Wessex Astrologer

Published in 2009 by
The Wessex Astrologer
4A Woodside Road
Bournemouth
BH5 2AZ
www.wessexastrologer.com

Oscar Hofman asserts the moral right to be recognised
as the author of this work.

ISBN 9781902405407
A catalogue record for this book is available at the British Library

Cover design by Dave at Creative Byte, Poole, Dorset.

Printed and bound in the UK by MPG Biddles Ltd, Kings Lynn, Norfolk,
England.

IMPORTANT NOTE

The information contained in this book is not intended to take the place of orthodox medical advice; it is given in the spirit of interest, and to promote further research. Certainly in the case of illness, advice should be sought from the proper medical authorities.

Contents

Preface

Part 1 The Basics

Chapter 1   The Humors and Elements in the Body   1
Chapter 2   Symptom and Disease   13
Chapter 3   Astrological Anatomy   18

Part 2 Diagnosis and Treatment

Chapter 4   Diagnosis: The Deeper Cause of Illness   27
Chapter 5   An Imbalance of Energy   50
Chapter 6   Cosmic Principles: Sympathy and Antipathy   59
Chapter 7   Treatment   66
Chapter 8   The Spiritual Level: Hildegard von Bingen   84
Chapter 9   Precious Stones   91

Part 3 Operations, Elections and Prevention

Chapter 10   Questions on Operations and Treatments   103
Chapter 11   Medical Elections   110
Chapter 12   Prevention   117

Appendix A - Stars Associated with Blindness   127
Appendix B - How to Spot Body Types   129
Epilogue   130
Glossary   133
Bibliography   136
Index   139

Preface - John Frawley

In 2006, I was keynote speaker at an astrological conference held in the medical school of Cape Town University. The conference was not associated with the university; the organisers had merely hired the lecture-halls for the weekend. During the conference, Rod Suskin, a first-magnitude star in the South African astrological firmament, told me that he had once been invited by the Medical School itself to lecture on the astrological approach to medicine.

The prospect had excited him. Speaking to medical students he could assume a basic knowledge of Galenic medical theory, so could quickly move on to advanced subjects. He was rapidly disabused of this idea, when his every mention of humours and temperament was met with blank stares of incomprehension. 'Haven't you been taught about Galen?' he asked. 'Only that his ideas are rubbish,' his audience replied. This instance of the tragic gulf between traditional and modern knowledge will surprise no one who has made even the briefest excursion into the history of science. Modern science seems able to exist without either historical or philosophical underpinning, much as a juggler's balls remain in the air without immediate support, and, because of this, often finds it necessary to gain credibility for itself by disparaging anything that went before. The science of the day before yesterday is nonsense, and anyone who practiced it must have been either a charlatan or a very foolish fellow.

Astrologers, who really should know better, seeing as their own forebears - simple-minded folk like Galileo and Kepler - are tarred with this brush, are eager to accept this principle as true. It is a commonplace in the world of modern astrology that 'death cannot be predicted from the birthchart because advances in modern medicine have extended the life-span'.

This idea does bring the comforting consequence that at some point in our life we can each expect to move beyond our fate, at which point we all get to marry Johnny Depp/Halle Berry (delete as applicable) and win the lotto every week. But it also carries the crazy implication that before the modern era medicine never extended anybody's life-span. Even the most basic of medical interventions, such as staunching a bleeding wound, never saved anyone's life.

Modern science, insofar as it condescends to pay any attention to its ancestors, sees them only in caricature: Columbus's sailors quivering on deck, waiting the moment when they would tumble from the edge of a flat world; the blood-letting physician, belabouring his patient with a machete, hoping only that he won't bleed to death before the bill is paid. As with the idea that our ancestors believed the earth to be flat, such medical myths abound.

The lack of pain-killers, for instance: palpably untrue, as is shown, for instance by Marcus Aurelius' physicians regulating his daily dosage of opium depending on how coherent he needed to be for that day's meetings. A delegation from Athens? Let him suffer. Some drunken Teutons? He could be wrecked and happy.

But it is not only the physicians of yore that the moderns so carelessly denigrate in their efforts to construct a facade of credibility around their own efforts to master the unmasterable art of restoring health; the patients too of olden days are criticised for believing that these quack remedies worked. Our ancestors were a remarkably silly lot. So when Moses Maimonides - surely one of the very last people who might be accused of either foolishness or charlatanry - is maintained as personal physician to the great Saladin, this must, it seems, be taken as proof of the latter's gullibility.

There have indeed been fools and incompetents in every age, but when the picture of traditional medicine painted for us by the moderns contains no characters but fools and incompetents, we might wonder how a picture of modern medicine based only on a week's worth of medical scandals drawn from our daily newspapers might appear. The image of traditional medicine that we are given draws mainly from the 18th century, which was probably the worst time in history to have fallen ill: the traditional wisdom had been shouldered aside, but the vacuum of knowledge thus created had not yet been filled with any of the 'magic bullets' of the moderns. Bullets which, it cannot be denied, can be of immediate efficacy, but which - it is hard to deny - by their failure to engage with the roots of the problem magic away the acute disorder in the present by trading it for chronic illness in the future.

An outcome more favourable to the shareholders of the pharmaceutical companies than it is to the populace in general.

We must, of course, avoid creating a rosy myth of the past: omnipotent physicians keeping a smiling populace in the pink of condition. Access to the best medical treatment was no more widespread then than it is today. But nor should this simple fact of logistics blind us to the merits of the traditional medical model: a model which concentrated on the patient as a whole, unified being, not on the symptoms as the product of an alien invading force.

Paul Starr's excellent *The Social Transformation of American Medicine*[1] describes the deliberate and concerted effort by doctors to improve and secure their social standing and income by removing medical knowledge from common provenance and turning it into an arcana scrutable only by the professional. He describes, for example, how D W Cathell's popular and oft-reprinted manual for medical practice, *The Physician Himself*, advises the doctor that 'by employing the terms ac. phenicum for carbolic acid, secale cornutum for ergot, kalium for potassium, natrum for sodium, chinin for quinia, etc., you will debar the average patient from reading your prescriptions.... You can also further eclipse his wisdom by transposing the terms'. [2]

The idea that illness could be attributed to a gang of invading aliens, germs, rather than to a lack of order within the body itself, proved a godsend for the doctors' cause. Here was their arcana delivered to them, shrouded in fogs far more impenetrable than the barrier of linguistic obscurity. These pesky varmints could not be seen nor their wily ways fathomed by any who had not been inducted into the cult. From within the laboratory, all previous medical knowledge was derided.

An early example of the physicians' effort to establish and maintain a monopoly over knowledge was the vitriol poured upon Nicholas Culpeper by the College of Physicians, when he dared to translate the *Pharmacopoeia* into the vernacular, with the intention of opening knowledge to the layman - the person, it must be remembered, who has the greatest interest in the body that is ill. This translation was denounced in press and pulpit, with accusations that he had mixed 'every receipt therein with some scruples, at least, of rebellion or atheism'.[3] While the exact wording of the denunciations has changed since then, no one who dares question the doctors' monopoly over medical knowledge

xii   Classical Medical Astrology

will be unfamiliar with the hysterical tones in which they are delivered. The author of the book you now hold might expect his ears to be similarly singed from certain quarters for daring to bridge the gulf in knowledge that consigns the traditional model of medicine to a safe quarantine in the distant past. As a worthy successor of Culpeper, Oscar Hofman is determined to present this knowledge not as a curiosity, a work of sterile intellectual archaeology, but as a living, practicable system that produces results.

As Culpeper proclaimed, paraphrasing Hippocrates, the very father of medicine, 'a physician without astrology is like a pudding without fat'.[4] So Oscar's approach to medical treatment is through astrology. It is apparent that the allopathic approach that dominates modern medicine has its failings. The human being is seen increasingly as a sophisticated piece of machinery, and the doctors, for all their increasing arrogance, increasingly relegate themselves to the role of mere mechanics. Of course, if the human being is no more than a piece of machinery, the cries to dispose of it as soon as it malfunctions cannot but be persuasive. But people are not machines; we differ. The most unsophisticated of car drivers is able to comprehend that putting petrol into a diesel engine is not wise. Yet the idea that people differ in their make-up in ways as fundamental as do varieties of internal combustion engine is, it seems, too complicated for the medical world to understand. The same drug should treat the same symptom in anyone; when it does not, the response is bafflement.

The astrological approach to diagnosis and prescription is inescapably holistic. What is treated is not a particular symptom, but a particular person in a particular state of disorder - of dis-ease - of which the symptom is a product. While the modern wonders why the drug that worked on person A quite fails on person B, despite their presenting identical symptoms, the traditional physician, precisely because they are person A and person B, does not expect them to react in the same way, no matter how similar their symptoms might appear. The use of astrology within the traditional medical model ensures that each treatment is personalised.

Of especial interest in Oscar's presentation of traditional astrological medicine is his integration of the work of Hildegard von Bingen, with its emphasis on the moral and spiritual causes of illness. The knee-jerk reaction from the sceptic to the idea that the person's moral and spiritual condition is causatively connected to their state of health is to ask if the chronically ill are really such great sinners, while those we see bouncing around the sportsfield in fine form are saints unrecognised, or to point out that saying three Hail Marys is not a cure-all. This reaction is to misunderstand. Job is not the only person who has been stricken with illness without it being a consequence of sinfulness. To accept that this connection exists is not at all to agree with that notorious England football manager whose daft theory was that those born disabled were suffering the consequences of lurid past lives. The suggestion here is not 'If thou sinnest, thou shalt break out in spots', but 'If thou dost break out in spots, the nature of those spots shalt be consequent upon the nature of thy sinfulness'.

What is claimed is that the human being, like the earth, has its fault-lines. Earthquakes do not have a random distribution across the earth's surface; they occur along the fault-lines. So with the human being: the illnesses suffered will be those congruent with the individual's personal fault-lines. A moment's reflection will demonstrate this, showing any of us that there are common ailments to which we have a propensity and other common ailments to which we are strangers. These fault-lines run deep. They are not contained solely in those superficial levels that manage our physical well-being. They extend to the very core of us, which is our soul. Hence the concept of sin cannot be ignored if the ailment is to be tackled at its root.

The knee-jerk dismissal of this idea rests on two assumptions, both of them superficial: one that sin is a rare occurrence, almost always committed by other people; the other, that illness is something that just should not happen, as if the patient could wave to a referee and appeal for an offside ruling against it. A wiser view would accept that both sin and illness are inevitable constituents of the human condition. The great theologian, Josef Pieper, draws the connection by playing on different meanings of the German word Heil. As his English translator explains, this 'is the standard theological term in German for salvation, while heilig means "holy" and is the standard prefix title for a saint. Unheil is equally generic and means any misalignment of that right functioning denoted by "health" and "whole", and can mean anything from nausea ("Ich fühle mich unheil") to a catastrophic disaster like an earthquake.'[5]

Sinfulness is a state of disorder; dis-ease is a state of disorder: the two states occurring in one person are congruent. This is why it is the centurion's plea over his sick servant that provides the words spoken immediately before receiving the soul's salvation: 'I am not worthy to receive you, but only say the word and I shall be healed'.

This does not, of course, mean that every time we get a cold we should head for the confessional. But the typical modern approach, with its emphasis on treating symptoms, is equivalent to locking up the person so he cannot sin. The traditional approach is more radical: it aims to change the person so he no longer inclines to sin. It aims to restore his healthy inner order, which will be reflected in a resolution of his dis-ease.

It is the inclusion of this material and its integration into a coherent system that elevates this book above a mere presentation of techniques of astrological medicine. Such would inevitably have fallen short of the great works of the past, as a translation must always fall short of the original. What Oscar Hofman has produced is an original, and one worthy to stand alongside any of the classic texts that stand as milestones along the highway of traditional knowledge. We may justly imagine their authors smiling down from whatever corner of heaven they now inhabit as they see they have a new peer.

I will end this brief introduction as I began it, with an anecdote. Some years ago I listened to a large number of doctors being interviewed on the effects of arthritis drugs. Doctor after doctor would discuss the latest products of the pharmaceutical industry, weighing their pros and cons. Then doctor after doctor would conclude that for all this constant innovation, the most effective treatment was one for which they had no explanation. It is, indeed, a treatment that sounds as if it has come straight from an alchemist's den: injections of gold. Perhaps those ancient physicians were not so foolish after all.

Notes

1. New York (?), 1982.
2. ibid. p.87.
3. *Mercurius Pragmaticus*, pt ii, no.21.
4. *Astrological Judgment of Diseases from the Decumbiture of the Sick*, London, 1655; rep. Nottingham, n.d., p.48.
5. *The Concept of Sin*, South Bend, 2001, p.52 and note.

PART ONE

THE BASICS

1

The Humors and Elements in the Body

Medical Astrology, A Seamless Unity

The four elements, Fire, Water, Earth and Air play a major part in medical classical astrology. These elements are the basic building-blocks of the whole cosmos, of which of course, our bodies are a part. Fire and Water, Earth and Air strongly influence all physical processes and therefore medical astrology always talks in terms of elements. The main parts of the medical consultation, diagnosis, prognosis and treatment can only be formulated and understood in these terms.

This is also the golden key which opens the treasure chest of medical astrology. Medical astrology consists of two parts: the astrological and the medical. By formulating in terms of elements these two parts are brought together as a matter of course, and because we can define everything in the cosmos in terms of Fire, Air, Water and Earth, there is no divide between the medical and the astrological components.

This distinguishes the classical approach from modern medical astrology, which does not integrate the astrological and medical parts so closely. What is usually called 'medical astrology' today is mostly naturopathy or homeopathy which is then loosely connected with charts. Sometimes a specific treatment is left out completely and only the psychological aspects are mentioned. The integral logical unity, with its many concrete possibilities for treatment, is not often found in these contemporary varieties of medical astrology.

The astrological elements are the building-blocks of our physical as well of our psychological functioning and we find them also in natural substances like herbs, precious stones and foodstuffs. This is the reason that a real astrological method of healing is possible. Everything is interconnected through the elements. In the past, up until the period we have given the strange name 'Enlightenment', a doctor was always an astrologer too. A doctor without astrological knowledge was seen as a blind man; a quack moving in the dark, who would probably hurt you rather than heal you.

From the Enlightenment onwards, traditional medicine incorporating astrology was rapidly discarded in favour of what has become our modern western medicine. Medical astrology was banned as a superstition and almost totally disappeared. It is only since the rebirth of astrology at the end of the nineteenth century in Theosophical circles in England, that charts and health have again been connected - and only now at the beginning of the 21st century is classical medical astrology returning to the place it deserves. This book seeks to be a contribution to this rehabilitation which will benefit the physical and mental health of so many people.

The Four Humors

In classical medical astrology the elements have special names, which will be used in the rest of this book. Fire is called yellow choler, Earth black choler, Water phlegm or slime and Air blood. These are the renowned humors or body fluids, for centuries the foundation of western traditional medicine based on the writings of the classical physicians Hippocratus and Galen. Before they start practising today, doctors still swear the Hippocratic Oath; one of the tiny traces of the tradition still found in modern medicine.

For an effective medical astrology, a thorough knowledge of the functions of the humors is essential. The four body fluids all have their specific functions and if a humor is not present in the required quantity, problems may result. To get a clear picture of the humors it is a good idea to think in specific images. What would be the result of an excess of the Fire element? An inflammation. It is that simple, although the humors can manifest in a very wide range of forms.

Although the elements or humors are the fundamental building-blocks of the cosmos they can be characterised in even more basic terms, the qualities. In modern astrology these have been largely forgotten but they are very important, certainly from a medical point of view. Every humor or element is a combination of two qualities which describe its temperature and its degree of moisture. Before the humors are discussed, we will first give some attention to the fundamental qualities.

Moisture and heat

The point of departure is a kind of creation myth: in the beginning there was heat. Heat is energy and life, it is impulse and motive. This is the first quality, the absolute though slightly abstract foundation of the material cosmos. Heat leads to movement and through movement energy is spent and things cool down. This is the second quality, coldness. This quality is based on the first impulse and has its origin in the absence of heat, which in turn makes things move. Coldness means that something does not function any more; there is not enough energy to keep processes going. This is the first axis. Heat and cold are the primary qualities.

The secondary qualities, moisture and dryness, develop out of the primary ones. If something cools down it will attract moisture; an object left outside overnight will become moist. If the sun rises and the temperature increases, we will soon see the fourth quality of dryness. It is not difficult to get a clear picture of the medical nature of these qualities. Because they are so closely connected to the elements their effects can be seen everywhere in nature and a medical astrologer can learn a lot simply by observing natural processes. What takes place in nature also takes place in the body, as outside so inside.

In this way the characteristics of the qualities can be specified further. Heat will move; it is energy and impulse. It also dries and will stimulate action. Cold will slow down and take out the energy. Moisture loses its form because it connects and softens. It will break down boundaries as one thing flows over into another and components are mixed. Dryness is its counterpart; it maintains form and closes itself off to create a clear boundary. These descriptions of qualities can be taken physically or psychologically; classical medical astrology does not distinguish sharply between those two levels of human functioning.

Yellow choler

The humors or elements can be built up out of these qualities in a logical way. Yellow choler, the choleric element, has the qualities of heat and dryness. So Fire has a high energy but it does not connect. It is heat which remains concentrated in a certain area, which is a clear picture of an inflammation, a typical yellow choler phenomenon. On a psychological level this is a fitting description of a Fire person, who will without much thinking, impulsively do what he thinks is right. The dryness in Fire means he will not connect; the heat gives him the high energy to act.

Too much yellow choler in the body will cause Fire phenomena, like the afore-mentioned inflammations, but fever and eczema are also typical examples as well as overactive organs like an overactive thyroid. An excess of a humor may lead to a great diversity of symptoms and diseases with the problem manifesting through the weakest point of the individual patient. Someone who has too much Fire can be recognized by general over-activity, a loud voice, a red dry skin and over-assertive behaviour.

The humors are also connected to the natural cycles, to the seasons. The yellow choler season is hot and dry; it is the summer, the second phase of the year. In the summer yellow choler diseases come to the fore and it is a good idea to adapt your diet to the season. An example is the Spanish *gazpacho*, a cold soup made of tomatoes and cucumbers, two moist and cooling vegetables. This dish is eaten a lot in summer in Andalusia, the hottest and most southerly part of Spain.

The physical-emotional developments in life can also be described in humoral terms. Yellow choler controls the second phase of puberty and adolescence. This is a Fire time when young people free themselves from the family and assert their independence. It is important that this Fire can leave the body through sports otherwise it may cause skin problems – the body will throw out excess heat through the skin. Fire also causes the typical teenage sexual obsessions – the term 'hot' was not invented for nothing. Too much yellow choler can be seen as a body ablaze.

In traditional physiology yellow choler has several functions. It thins the blood so it will be able to reach the smallest capillaries everywhere in the body. Yellow choler is used for building up tissues like lung tissue and muscles. This sharp fiery humor is stored in the gall bladder and used to clean the intestines. Fire is also connected to the heart as the organ of the spontaneous first impulse. It is clear that all these functions may become disturbed if there is too much or not enough yellow choler.

Phlegm or slime

The opposite of yellow choler is phlegm, also referred to as slime or Water. Water is characterised by coldness and moisture and it will, if it is present in excess, cause slime-like phenomena – processes that become too fluid, lacking in form. Good examples of so-called Water diseases are colds, flu, bronchitis and sinusitis, though it may also manifest as diarrhoea or even as psoriasis or dementia. How phlegm looks in a more material form will become clear if you have a bad cold. Because phlegm is the element of emotions, an excess of slime may be connected to grief or apathy.

Phlegm is cold and moist so it has little energy, but it does have the capacity to connect. This also describes on a psychological level the phlegmatic person; one who has strong emotions but is not very active by nature; one who has intense emotional and intimate relations with others, often with family members. So the psychological and physical effects of connecting and a lack of energy are similar. The two levels are interwoven and this relationship can be described precisely by the humors.

The key words for phlegm are 'cooling', 'streaming along' and 'a lack of form'. Water streaming down from the mountains through a river-bed is a good image. The water will follow the river-bed unless there is too much water, then the river will flood and damage other fixed forms because of its own lack of form. Too much phlegm can be seen as an inundation of the body.

People who have too much phlegm can be recognized by their passiveness, their pale moist skin, their timid behaviour and soft voice. They do not have the Fire to take action and fight for their interests. The lack of form means that phlegm will stay attached and stick, in both a psychological and a physical sense. A nice example is the moist fingertip used for turning pages – the moisture sticks to the page so you can turn it, if it is dry you cannot: moisture connects.

The physiological function of phlegm can easily be described as a general lubricant. Moisture is needed to make things run smoothly; imagine what will happen if joints dry out. The cold and moist Water also acts as a counterpart to hot and dry yellow choler and prevents over-heating of the body. Because of its streaming nature it is responsible for excretion and expulsion and it produces saliva, lymph fluids and mucous membranes. It is stored in the lungs making them sensitive to phlegmatic diseases. Slime is also connected to the kidney function.

Phlegm is the humor of winter, so it is important to eat more hot and dry foods in winter to compensate for the moisture and cold of the season. In life, phlegm dominates the very last phase and this soft sensitive humor can be seen in the typical mildness of old people or as the typical spitting old man. Dementia is another phlegm phenomenon; the formless slime undermines the clearly delineated mental processes and this is a danger, especially for people with a phlegmatic constitution. Changes in the diet may work preventively against dementia.

A special phlegmatic phase in life is pregnancy. This is the largest-scale process of expulsion imaginable and therefore we need some slime here. It explains the typical psychological and physical phenomena in pregnancy: the over-sensitivity, the strange appetite so difficult to control, the lack of iron, (iron as a fiery Mars metal is connected to the counterpart of phlegm: yellow choler), the instability of the pelvis – these are all signs of weakening caused by the excess of phlegm in the body. The pregnant female body is also a clear physical example of phlegm: its roundness, its lack of form, the moisture present everywhere. It shows how phlegm can manifest.

Because phlegm is the body fluid of feeling, the moisture balance has a direct impact on our emotional stability. Many people do not drink enough water and this may cause emotional imbalance. Phlegm streams and we need this streaming, as it clears toxins from our bodies - a normal part of daily life. The first step towards a more stable emotional life is to take in enough moisture, for a standard adult that is about two litres a day. This will create a basis for a healthier emotional state.

Naturally there is a mutual exchange here. The physical level influences the psychological level but the psyche also touches the body. Grief which is not expressed may become stuck as tears that were not cried and will increase the amount of phlegm in the body. Psychological and physical are no more than terms describing two ways in which the humors may manifest in the human system. The psyche is, as it were, the thinner, less material version of the body. There are other factors which play a role, as for example spiritual factors, and these will be discussed in Chapter 8 about Hildegard von Bingen.

YELLOW CHOLER

heat   dryness

BLOOD   BLACK

moisture   cold

PHLEGM

Figure 1. Humors and qualities
Humors consist of two qualities: yellow choler for example is hot and
dry.

Blood
The third, sanguine humor is blood, the element of life. Blood is hot and
moist, it gives energy which remains connected, and this is a suitable
image of the life process itself. Nevertheless an excess of blood will cause
diseases, possibly in the heart and the circulatory system, though it may
also lead to nervousness, exhaustion, migraine and bleedings. In fact
these are attempts of the body to correct itself by initiating spontaneous
bloodletting. An excess of blood may lead to an increased vulnerability
to infection; by its moist nature blood decreases the innate heat which
can undermine the immune system.

Heat and moisture gives a combination of energy and the capacity
to connect, which is the picture of the social and friendly character of the
typical Air person. Moisture wants to contact others and the heat leads
to activity; this is the good-humoured communicative sanguine type.
The nature of blood is expansive and a sanguine person likes to have a
lot of contacts, some of which will be rather superficial because sanguine
people also love movement. This image can be seen in the activity of the
blood in our bodies, it travels to all parts of the organism, it exchanges
substances, it brings nutrients and carries off waste products. The liver
is the organ where the blood is stored.

Apart from forming the red fluid in our bodies, blood also has
an important role in the digestion of foods; its warm and moist energy

breaks down foods in the stomach and in the liver. Blood provides the brain and heart with energy and builds up sperm and mother's milk. Blood is clearly connected to fertility. It has an expansive character and blood diseases can be compared to a hot vapour, a kind of steam in the body.

The blood season is spring, when everything starts to grow and bud. There is still enough moisture present, the summer heat has not yet dried it up, so there is still a good balance. In terms of the phase of life, this represents youth. The cheerful playfulness of children, their careless expansive behaviour so difficult to discipline, seamlessly fits the energetic nature of the sanguine humour. In this blood phase there is an increased danger of infection, which manifests as the well-known childhood diseases.

Melancholy or black choler
The counterpart of happy blood is the melancholic humor or black choler. This is cold and dry and is the most dangerous of all the humors because it is opposed to the warm and moist nature of life. Cold and dryness give us a combination of low energy without connection, an image of processes becoming rigid. Melancholy typically leads to diseases with broken connections and energy drained off. Examples are multiple sclerosis, depressions, Parkinson's disease and constipation.

Melancholy gives a pale colour like phlegm, but it looks drier and emaciated. Phlegm still wants to connect, black choler isolates and breaks off contacts. This is the typical melancholy depression which cannot see any point in life any more, in contrast to the phlegmatic 'depression' which is more like grief and is caused by stuck emotions. People with a lot of black choler in their constitution are often thin and long and can be recognized by their laconic behaviour. These kinds of people are more vulnerable to depression because they naturally have a lot of black choler in their body-mind systems.

In traditional physiology black choler does have several very important functions. All hard parts of the body are built up out of black choler such as hair, bones and nails. Black choler has a slowing effect and it is important in the digestive process because it holds foods long enough to be properly digested. It gives fixedness and firmness and psychologically perseverance and discipline. Black choler is stored in the spleen, and can be sent from there to the stomach to create appetite. It is a signal to the stomach that food is needed when the body becomes cold and dry.

In the cycle of the seasons, the melancholic humor is connected to autumn with its falling leaves and the processes of nature slowing down. For those who are vulnerable to this, depression looms at this time and more warm and moist sanguine foods can compensate the excess black choler to prevent the typical autumn dip. The melancholic phase in life is adulthood, often a contrast to our more carefree childhood.

In this phase from about age 40 to 60 responsibilities are often heavy, the career is nearing its summit while at the same time children are growing up and our parents may need care. One has to work and the limitations inherent in life have to be accepted. Vital energy is decreasing; going out all night is not possible any more and the first physical limitations have to be accepted. This is the phase of continuation and concrete duties, an image which fits black choler. Socially it is not the most abundant period as dryness cuts off connections, psychologically as well as medically.

The humors in their several aspects are the most basic building-blocks of classical medical astrology. They describe the medical, social and psychological functioning of man and they give a picture of the nature of the seasons and the phases of life. They also show what can go wrong if the balance between the humors is disturbed and an illness develops. The nature of the illness can be characterized by the nature of the afflicting humor and on this healing measures can be based. In Chapters 4 and 5 practical diagnosis and treatment will be discussed.

Four or five elements?

This book is very much focused on practical issues, and it is possible to work effectively with a division into four humors in combination with the chart as a diagnostic tool. A medical astrologer working with the humoral model will be able to bring healing even in cases given up by whole teams of specialists. So we are using a powerful model in this book, but there is more. Those who have some knowledge of eastern healing methods such as Ayurvedic medicine or traditional Chinese medicine know these models use five elements, although Ayurvedic medicine reduces this to only three 'doshas' in practice.

This may seem to contradict the western humoral model, but it does not. In some western approaches there is a fifth element on a higher level called the quintessence or the ether. The ether is an element of a more subtle, finer substance and in it the other four coarser elements have their origin. The fifth element is the connective medium to the higher, non-material world; the planetary forces project themselves through the ether into matter. It describes the phase of the formation of ideas which can realise themselves later in the matter of the four coarse humors.

The ether has hardly any direct humoral effects in the sense of cooling, heating, drying or moistening, it is the finer, etheric element. However it does connect to the higher worlds and is always involved to some degree. It would be too materialistic a view to see human beings as mere mixtures of four coarse humors; it is the ether that makes the difference. The fifth etheric element is closest to Air and is therefore connected to the Air planet Jupiter and the liver, the ultimate Jupiter organ.

It is important to keep the ether in mind. Although we can work effectively with the four coarse humors, man is more than coarse matter. The model of the five elements could be seen as the background theory to the model of the four humors. It shows there are more influences on health and disease than just coarse and material factors. So the model of the four humors does not contradict the theory of the five elements; on the contrary it is a part of it. The model of the four humors will be central in medical astrology, although in practical terms other factors will also be discussed at some points.

2

Symptom and Disease

Materialistic vision

The relationship between modern and traditional medicine is characterized by the difference between the ancient spiritual and cosmic vision of life and Enlightenment materialism. The present-day scientifically based view of the world depends on that which can be seen, touched and measured. Modern hospitals invest in advanced diagnostic devices which can reveal health problems long before they would usually be detected, but this can lead to the patient being seen as a collection of individual symptoms; the view taken by traditional medicine is that the symptom is merely the final result of something which lies much deeper in the human physical-psychological organism.

One of the drawbacks with the sophisticated drugs used in modern medicine is that they can often relieve the symptoms without curing the cause, so the symptoms will re-appear at a later date. Traditional medicine views the client holistically so that any imbalance can be corrected at a very deep level before it has the chance to become more serious.

Modern medicine's preference to observe what is happening on the material level and try to fight the symptoms presented is a logical consequence of the philosophy out of which scientific medicine has progressed: the rationalistic and materialistic vision of 17th century Enlightenment. This development was a break with the past; the first signs showing up during the Renaissance. In those days the spiritual and cosmic perspective started to shift gradually towards the worldly, the personal and the material.

The Renaissance is the decisive development in western culture, because it was at this point that the dominantly spiritual traditional orientation was abandoned. This change of perspective, and the

Enlightenment which is its radical consequence, is indicated astrologically by the precessional ingress of important fixed stars into new signs and by the Great Conjunction of Jupiter and Saturn on 18 December 1603. For the first time in more than eight centuries, the cycle of the Great Conjunctions began again in a Fire sign, in Sagittarius. In traditional mundane astrology this indicates the disappearance of the dominant religion and the rise of another vision of life, in this case the materialistic philosophy or, better, 'religion' of science.

Many symptoms, four causes

In traditional medicine we look further than symptoms - in fact there are only four kinds of diseases: Earth, Water, Air and Fire diseases. Our bodies are part of the cosmos and the cosmos is built up of the four basic energies of the elements, it is that simple. Disease in the traditional approach is always a disturbance of the balance between the four humors or elements. One of the four humors is present in excess and this excess has to be dealt with.

These four basic causes can manifest in many different ways in the human organism. The same symptom might even be caused by different humors in excess, or an excess of the same humour may cause different symptomatic images. In the traditional approach there is a complex and subtle relationship between the deeper real cause of the disease and the symptom as the surface manifestation of the unbalanced state. So there is no direct, linear relationship here between symptom and disease. The symptoms on the outside do not necessarily make clear what the real cause of the problem is. A good example is eczema, which dermatology doesn't treat very effectively. Superficially, eczema is most often a Fire phenomenon; yellow choler comes out through the skin. But this does not mean that a yellow choler excess is also the cause of the problem.

Practice shows that skin diseases may be caused by different kinds of humors in excess. It could be yellow choler, but it might just as well be phlegm, blood or sometimes even black choler. If yellow choler is the cause, the Fire excess is let out through the skin, leading to the typical red fiery spots or sometimes inflammation if there is a really large excess. But if phlegm is the cause, Fire also comes out through the skin, but in this case the organism has become so enormously watery that it does not 'know' what to do with the Fire in the body and simply throws it out.

So the same disease may be caused by different humors; in fact these are different diseases manifesting in the same way. It also applies to our common diseases such as heart problems, high blood-pressure and cancer. Scientific medicine treats these problems differently. A good example is cortisone which is often prescribed for eczema. Cortisone is cold and it cools Fire very effectively but this is a superficial effect. This toxic substance may cause problems in other parts of the body because it cools too much. In the longer term, lung problems may develop if this organ, which is very sensitive to slime formation, becomes too cold; too much phlegm is produced and the result may be chronic asthma or bronchitis.

It will be clear that if the real cause of the eczema is moist and cold phlegm excess (as is often the case) the cortisone will have an extra damaging effect. The cold condition which has led to the fiery eczema is worsened by the cold medication. Although the Fire phenomenon on the outside is cooled off somewhat, the pathogenic cold condition of the body is aggravated. In the longer term this will lead to a chronic problem which will often be treated with further cooling measures.

The same thing applies to cancer, which is a symptom, its deeper cause being an excess of one of the four humours. Again we see that different causes lead to more or less the same symptom, cancer being an alarm-bell that something is seriously out of order. It is mostly treated with cool and dry medication in modern medicine to limit the proliferation of cells, but this will have a damaging effect if the deeper cause is black choler (which often is the case). Black choler is cold and dry and the side-effect of the medication is that the excess of black choler will increase further. The symptom is suppressed temporarily but the deeper cause remains, which is the reason that cancer often returns.

Fortunately modern treatment is sometimes successful, in which case the deeper cause is mostly too much heat and the cooling medication will then have a positive effect on the symptom and the deeper cause.

A cooperation between traditional and modern doctors could be extremely fruitful. The astrologer can see what the deeper cause of the illness is in terms of heat/cold/dryness/moisture and this diagnosis could be used in the treatment. Classical medical astrologers are able to look behind the screen of superficial reality because they use charts; astrology reduces phenomena to their real causes because it has knowledge of the structure of the cosmos. There are not more than four building-blocks – Fire, Water, Earth and Air – and seven dynamic forces, the planets, which move everything. This principle can be applied to the whole cosmos and even an astrologer without any medical training can prescribe effective remedies against many diseases.

Blood-letting?

A fine illustration of the scientific attitude in schools and universities towards the traditional approach is blood-letting. Most of us will immediately see an image of an old-fashioned quack with big, round glasses, watching his patient bleeding to death without doing anything. According to modern convictions this was a horrible form of superstition which claimed many, many victims. This is totally untrue and is an image deliberately created to ridicule the tradition; it is not based on fact at all.

Blood-letting was a method which was always applied with much care. Firstly, small quantities of blood were let out, mostly not more than 150 ml. In modern medical practice a blood donor gives much more, often half a litre. Secondly, the blood-letting was always carefully prepared and the patient had to subject himself to a special regimen for several days, both before and after the treatment. Thirdly, the whole process was timed astrologically and the patient had to meet very strict conditions. He could not have a blood-letting if he was too weak. Under the correct circumstances blood-letting is a very effective measure preventively or as part of a treatment.

Infectious diseases

A modern day obsession of modern medicine is germs, bacteria and viruses. Many diseases are reduced to germs entering the body. To a certain extent this is true, although it depends on the level you are thinking. It is undeniable that germs have their role in causing diseases and that killing them by antibiotics or anti-viral medication may make sense and may be effective. But there is more to this. A person who is humorally balanced will not be infected so easily; if the body is well-balanced it will resist the infecting germs and render them harmless. Secondly, infections can be treated very well on the humoral level. If the humoral balance is restored, the germs will disappear. So we have a difference in the level of approach here. The traditional treatment will first restore the balance, as a result of which the body itself can deal with the germs; modern medicine works on the premise that the germs must be destroyed. In this case the body has not had a chance to correct the imbalance or develop a resistance and the infection may return.

3

Astrological Anatomy

Signs, houses and body parts

Now that we have discussed the way the humors work, and the relation between symptoms and the cause of the disease, we only need one other building-block for an effective medical astrology: astrological anatomy. Astrological symbolism describes the body through the houses, the planets and the signs. Signs and houses refer to body parts in a purely anatomical way, so Leo and the fifth house describe the heart. Astrological anatomy is the only field in traditional astrology in which houses and signs are interpreted in more or less the same way; this parallel so widely used in modern astrology is not found anywhere else in classical astrology.

The image which illustrates this symbolism is a human figure encircling the chart. The head starts with Aries and the figure ends with the feet in Pisces. The same can be shown for the houses, the first house will describe the head and the twelfth house the feet. In practice the anatomy by houses is used more often. To check the condition of the liver, we first look at the fifth house and its ruler in the chart and at planets which might be present in the fifth house.

These anatomical systems are to be used with a considerable degree of flexibility and pragmatism. There is not one approach which is always right; sometimes it is the house which gives the clearest indication, sometimes the sign and sometimes the planet. To determine the anatomical location of the disease we can use the following guidelines:

Aries/1st house	Head
Taurus/2nd house	Neck, throat
Gemini/3rd house	Hands, arms, shoulders
Cancer/4th house	Breast, lungs
Leo/5th house	Heart, liver, stomach, back, sides

Virgo/6th house	Intestines, bowels, belly
Libra/7th house	Urinary/reproductive system, lower back
Scorpio/8th house	Organs of excretion, anus
Sagittarius/9th house	Hips, buttocks
Capricorn/10th house	Knees
Aquarius/11th house	Calves, ankles
Pisces/12th house	Feet

The scheme is based mainly on the anatomical place in the body, so there may be a certain overlap. This is the reason why some organs are attributed to more than one house. Also the parallel between signs and houses is not perfect. Genitals are given to Scorpio but also to the seventh house. Of course genitals and organs of excretion are close, but Scorpio and the eighth house seem to describe the external parts.

The first house is of particular importance as it not only describes the limited region of the head, but also the body as a whole. This is the key to astrological diagnosis, which will be discussed further in Chapters 4 and 5. The traditional authorities do not agree on all the attributions, especially if the bladder, the kidneys and the genitals are concerned. But astrology is always logical, so we can be encouraged to think for ourselves and try to see the principle behind it.

The opposition can be especially clarifying. The second house is connected to the throat and food, and everything that is used to maintain the body. It refers to the resources a person has at his disposal, the things that support him in his battle for survival. So in the opposite house we will find what belongs to others and all that goes out; therefore the organs of excretion. This also applies to the seventh house which is concerned with others and relationships, and so we find the reproductive system here.

The kidneys are a difficult case, as they are sometimes given to the sixth house, sometimes to the seventh house. But as they are associated with Libra and involved so clearly in the urinary system, it is a good idea to give them to the seventh house. Because so many organs are attributed to houses 5 to 8, it can be a little unclear, but with some creativity and flexibility the system works well in practice, all the more so because we mainly work with specific horary questions.

Practice has shown that there is no detailed correspondence between very specific parts of human anatomy and certain zodiacal degrees. There is no degree which very specifically refers to one vertebra or one small specific part of the intestines. What does work is the division of the signs on a house. Suppose we have Libra on the first part of the ninth house and Scorpio on the second. In that case the first sign will describe the buttocks and the second sign the hips. The condition of Libra's ruler Venus shows the state of the buttocks and the condition of Mars, Scorpio's ruler, the state of the hips.

Planets and organs

Not only the houses and the signs but also the planets have an anatomical meaning. To understand this it is important to have a clear idea of the function of the planets in the chart. In traditional astrology the signs are only the background against which the planets work, whereas the planets are the dynamic forces which act and make things move. The characteristics ascribed to the signs by modern astrology used to belong to the planets which rule these signs. The reason they 'rule' at all is exactly that they are the forces that shape and move things, they can act. The typical description of Libra in modern astrology is a classical description of Venus, Libra's ruler.

This misconception has clouded many things that were once clear in astrology. A sign is not a house and a planet is not the same as a sign. Planets work at another more tangible, active level than signs. They represent the seven dynamic forces which shape our world. Medically the seven planets are seven energy streams in the body which take concrete shape in different organs. The planetary energy streams are reflected in the function of the organs. To show how this principle works in practice we can consider the organs given to Saturn. These are the bladder, the skin, the teeth, the bones and joints, the spleen and the right ear. The skin is the boundary with the outside world and the demarcation of the body, a very Saturnian function. Bones are the framework providing structure and firmness; the bladder is the keeper of moisture; the spleen stores and processes black choler, the humour that corresponds to the cold and dryness of Saturn. The immune system also falls under Saturn. It is like a second skin which guards the boundary with the outside world.

The symbolism of the right ear is a bit unclear. It probably originates in the traditional attribution of hearing to Saturn. It is the right ear because the right organ in a pair is always seen as the most important organ, and so it receives the planet for the general function. If it is necessary to make that distinction, the other member of the pair is allocated another planet; in this case the left ear comes under Mars traditionally. I cannot see why though.

Jupiter is the Great Benefic in classical astrology and refers to the liver, the lungs, the cartilage and the sperm. The liver is the great detoxifying organ, warm and moist, and the central post which forms and divides the humours through the body and so makes life possible. The lungs are clearly connected with Air and Jupiter is the Airy planet. Jupiter is also moist which describes the cartilage, which is firm but soft, not as hard as the Saturnal bones. It is a connective tissue of an elastic nature, a kind of soft, moist form of the real bone.

Mars is not only the left ear, it is also the bile, the sharp fluid which attacks and breaks down fats and is used to clean the intestines. It also symbolizes iron in the body and blood, but only in connection with wounds if found outside the body. The quality of the blood itself is given by Jupiter, whereas the blood circulation as a function is connected to the heart, and is described by the Sun which symbolizes the heart. Mars also represents the genitals, especially the male sexual organs. This planet also has a role in the immune system.

It is logical that the Sun, the Great Light, refers to seeing and the eyes, specifically the right eye in men and the left eye in women. Again we have a remarkable symbolism of right and left, and in this case it has been checked in practice: it absolutely works. The Sun is the head and the brain, in its function as the central commanding and coordination post for the whole body. The Sun is the leader and the king, the centre which initiates activity. It shows that we need the vital solar energy to make the central nervous system work well.

Venus clearly is associated with the (female) genitals and with the kidneys which maintain the moisture balance and are also cold and moist like the planet itself. She also refers to the throat.

Mercury is the nervous system, thinking and imagination, the fingers, the hands and the tongue. It also refers to the head but not in the same way as the Sun. Mercury is concerned with passing the message, purely the connective aspect, not with the central coordinating function.

Sometimes Mercury is associated with the lungs, but this seems to refer more to the aspect of exchange of waste products and air and to its antipathy to Jupiter. The Airy Great Benefic certainly describes the lungs in general better than cold and dry Mercury.

Finally the Moon as the moist and cold mother planet refers to the bladder, the womb, the breasts, the belly and the intestines (the Moon as the flushing function). It symbolizes the left eye in men and the right eye in women. The Moon is also associated with the brain and the head, as the counter-part of Mercury. Mercury is rational thinking and the Moon is the other half of the brain with a more emotional, intuitive function.

It will be clear that this astrological connection of planet functions to organs has some advantages compared to the signs/houses system. If the astrologer wants to check the condition of the immune system in the context of a question, Saturn will be the right significator. Also Mercury as the general significator of the nervous system and rational thinking can often be of use. There is even a fourth system of anatomical symbolism which uses the planet-in-sign position as a whole. This system can be used to find the anatomical place affected by the disease and it is given below (taken from Lilly's *Christian Astrology* Book 1).

In Aries
Saturn: breast/arms; Jupiter: neck/throat/heart/belly; Mars: belly/head; Sun: thighs; Venus; kidneys/feet; Mercury: genitals/legs; Moon: knees/head.

In Taurus
Saturn: heart/breast/belly; Jupiter: shoulders/arms/belly/neck; Mars: kidneys/throat; Sun: knees; Venus: genitals/head; Mercury: thighs/feet; Moon: legs/throat.

In Gemini
Saturn: belly/heart; Jupiter: breast/reins/genitals; Mars: genitals/arms/breast; Sun: legs/ankles; Venus: thighs/throat; Mercury: knees/head; Moon: feet/shoulders/arms/thighs.

In Cancer
Saturn: kidneys/belly/genitals; Jupiter: heart/genitals/thighs; Mars:

heart/breast/thighs; Sun: feet; Venus: knees/shoulders/arms; Mercury: legs/throat/eyes; Moon; head/breast/stomach.

In Leo
Saturn: genitals/kidneys; Jupiter: belly/thighs/knees; Mars: knees/heart/belly; Sun: head; Venus: legs/breast/heart; Mercury: feet/arms/shoulders/throat; Moon: throat/stomach/heart.

In Virgo
Saturn: thighs/genitals/feet; Jupiter: kidneys/knees; Mars: legs/belly; Sun: throat; Venus: feet/stomach/heart/belly; Mercury: head/breast/heart; Moon: arms/shoulders/bowels.

In Libra
Saturn: knees/thighs; Jupiter: genitals/legs/head/eyes; Mars: feet/reins/genitals; Sun: shoulders/arms; Venus: head/small guts; Mercury: throat/heart/stomach/belly; Moon: breast/kidneys/heart/belly.

In Scorpio
Saturn: knees/legs; Jupiter: thighs/feet; Mars: head/genitals/arms/thighs; Sun: breast/heart; Venus: throat/kidneys/genitals; Mercury: shoulders/arms/bowels/back; Moon: stomach/heart/genitals/belly.

In Sagittarius
Saturn: legs/feet; Jupiter: knees/head/thighs; Mars: throat/thighs/hand/feet; Sun: heart/belly; Venus: shoulders/arms/genitals/thighs; Mercury: breast/kidneys/heart/genitals; Moon: bowels/thighs/back.

In Capricorn
Saturn: head/feet; Jupiter: neck/legs/knees/eyes; Mars: arms/shoulders/knees/legs; Sun: belly/back; Venus: breast/heart/thighs; Mercury: stomach/heart/genitals; Moon: kidneys/knees/thighs.

In Aquarius
Saturn: neck/head; Jupiter: feet/arms/shoulders/breast; Mars: breast/legs/heart; Sun: kidneys/genitals; Venus: heart/knees; Mercury: bowels/thighs/heart; Moon: genitals/legs/ankles.

In Pisces
Saturn: arms/shoulders/neck; Jupiter: head/breast/heart; Mars: heart/feet/belly/ankles; Sun: genitals/thighs; Venus: belly/legs/neck/throat; Mercury: kidneys/knees/genitals/thighs; Moon: thighs/feet.

The planets are seen as dynamic energy streams in the body. The seven streams determine the physical, mental and psychological functions, but always against a background of the humoral balance. It depends a lot on the sign a planet is placed in as to whether it will be able to manifest in an effective and balanced way. If the humoral nature of the sign (hot/cold/moist/dry) is not the same as the nature of a planet, this causes disease. In the next chapter we will consider how we can diagnose on the basis of the horary chart and this principle.

In this whole scheme the outer planets have only a minor role. They are not seen as real planets, but rather as a special category of fixed stars. They are only important if a relevant planet narrowly aspects an outer planet, and this is always unfavourable. Outer planets do not rule signs and so they cannot be taken as house rulers. They do not really symbolize an energy stream in the body organs, nor any other functions, so they are only taken into consideration when they have a meaningful role to fulfil.

Hormonal glands
There is a remarkable parallel between the planets as the seven dynamic forces of creation and the seven most important glands in the body. Glands are pre-eminently the contact points between psyche and body and they have an important overall regulating function in the human body/mind system. The seven planetary forces are expressed in these glands, and they are the points at which the planets very clearly touch the human organism. In top-down order these most important glands are: pineal gland, pituitary gland, thyroid gland, thymus, pancreas, adrenal glands and sexual glands.

The pineal gland is seen as the seat of the soul, it occupies the highest position closest to 'heaven'. This gland produces hormones which suppress the activity of the sexual glands until puberty, a very Saturnian function. We can see that Saturn's role as a boundary planet, the guardian on the threshold of the divine dimension, is relevant in the spiritual meaning often given to the pineal gland. It is further closely connected to the regulation of the biological clock and time rhythms. The pineal gland produces melatonin – melan = black = Saturn – a substance that strengthens the immune system, increases the quantity of 'killer cells' and stimulates the growth of bone marrow cells. All Saturnian things. Most strikingly, the crystals apatite and calcite are found in the pineal gland; minerals connected to the Moon/Saturn axis.

According to Galen, one of the founding fathers of humoral medicine, one of the most important functions of the pineal gland was controlling the movements of the *pneuma*. The pneuma is seen as a kind of spiritual stream of 'air' very strongly connected to higher dimensions and the source of vital energy. Pneuma is more or less the same as prana, the spiritual energy in Ayurvedic medicine. The pneuma is taken into the body by breathing; the pineal gland with its Saturn nature grounds it. The pineal gland is also associated with the third eye, which refers to its spiritual nature.

The pituitary gland is the Jupiter energy and it has a central regulating role in the whole system of glands. The Sun is the king but Jupiter represents the aristocracy, the governing elite, and this manifests clearly in the function of this gland. It coordinates and integrates the many growth processes; it has the typical jovial "long term" vision on the physical level. Next, the thyroid gland produces heat and therefore energy through processes of decomposition, a clear martial symbolism. It is the only gland that needs iodine, a sharp corrosive substance of a martial nature, to function well.

The fourth gland, the thymus, is close to the heart and was seen as useless for a long time. However removing the thymus leads to a general decrease of vitality, growth power and resistance of the whole system, so it clearly incorporates a solar symbolism. As we get older it degenerates further and further, mirroring the loss of vital energies. The fifth gland, the pancreas, is associated with the sugar level and maintaining the right balance, which points to its Venus nature.

The next gland has in many aspects a double function, producing adrenalin and noradrenalin to give the alertness to react adequately to threats in the environment. It creates a clear and sharp mercurial connection with what surrounds us. Typically the adrenal glands occur as a pair; doubling is a mercurial theme. The adrenal cortex also connects interweaves with the nervous system, which is also mercurial.

Finally, the sex glands are connected with reproduction, in which we see the lunar aspect of motherhood and fertility. It will be clear that this gland can also be associated with strong emotions and desires. Through the Moon, the planet closest to Earth, which indicates spontaneous emotional impulses and earth-bound longings, the hunger for life is expressed very strongly in the possibility of reproduction. It is striking that we find the antipathy between Saturn and Moon also on the glandular level, as the pineal gland will suppress the sexual glands till puberty.

This can also be seen in the complementary/opposing roles of Mars and Venus in the thyroid glands and the pancreas. The thyroid gland regulates the production of heat, while the pancreas maintains the right level of raw materials for this process. These are two aspects of the same process. The mercurial adrenals give immediate alertness, which is the counter-part of the jovial-pituitary long-term growth and "planning". As the solar gland, the thymus occupies a central balancing and vitalising place. The anatomical position of the glands mirrors the planetary axis formation; the pineal gland is for example the highest gland and the lunar sexual glands have the lowest position.

PART TWO

DIAGNOSIS

AND

TREATMENT

4

Diagnosis:
The Deeper Cause of Illness

Horaries

Modern astrology always focuses strongly on the natal chart, whereas in classical astrology the emphasis is more on horary charts. We can only base reliable treatment and diagnosis on the chart of a question about the disease. This can not be done by the natal chart, which is almost solely used to give preventive advice. The reason for this is quite simple. A horary chart of a question about a medical situation always shows the condition of the client at that moment very clearly. In a natal chart we cannot be too sure about what we see.

Horary charts are also better for this purpose because in practice a medical astrologer will receive many questions from patients suffering from chronic illnesses. Progressions or transits active at the moment of the consultation do not show the problem so unambiguously. Chronic diseases which have existed for years may sometimes be mirrored in progressions many years before the consultation, but in most cases this too is unclear. The progression that led to the development of the disease and the kind of disturbance this caused in the body cannot be seen in the natal chart with the precision required.

Moreover, dietary habits, life style, the psychological condition and medical treatments strongly influence the physical balance in the body. You never know exactly how a person has lived and what has happened. These are choices people are free to make in their lives and they cannot be read in the natal chart. You cannot base reliable diagnoses and treatment on the necessarily incomplete life story of the client in combination with his natal chart. Therefore most modern medical astrologers do not diagnose or treat but limit themselves to general psychological advice, or else they are homeopaths or natural healers who may use the chart as a quick reference in conjunction with other therapies.

Horary charts can be used as a reliable instrument for diagnosis and treatment, and all that is needed is a thorough understanding of astrology, of the functions of the humors and of the method of analysis itself. The treatment advice based on a horary analysis is not too complicated to draw up but it will help of course if you are a naturopath. Astromedical practice can be compared to a certain extent with other forms of healing which do not use astrology. Examples are Ayurvedic medicine, Unani Tibb (Islamic humoral medicine in southern Asia) and TCM – Traditional Chinese Medicine. These approaches use a similar model in which heat, moisture and the elements play the main parts, although diagnosis takes place by detailed observation; for example of the tongue, the pulse, the urine, the faeces and the skin. An experienced Chinese or Unani doctor will be able to see which humor is in excess without looking at a chart.

The medicine of the humors as used in medical astrology has been preserved in its purest form in Unani medicine, which is relatively unknown in the western world. Unani is widely practised in southern Asia, for example in India and Pakistan, and is much supported by the government in India as a cheap and effective form of health care. Whereas Unani is strongly associated with Islam, the local Ayurvedic medicine has its roots in Hinduism. In fact Unani has Greek origins, the word 'Unani' means Ionic. In Unani Tibb traditional western medicine is still alive and kicking, so we can also use Unani remedies in classical medical astrology.

Dignity

To be able to diagnose reliably by means of classical medical astrology you need to know the classical system of dignities. There are two kinds of dignities describing two kinds of power. The first dignity is essential dignity. The level of essential dignity is assessed by a planet's position in a sign. Mars in Aries is in its own sign and therefore has a lot of essential dignity. But Mars is also strong in Capricorn where it has its exaltation.

There are also negative counterparts of a placement of a planet in its own sign or in exaltation, called detriment and fall respectively. If a planet is placed in a negative dignity it cannot do much good and is then essentially debilitated. An example is Mars in Libra. Placed opposite to its own sign, it is in detriment there; a bad Mars which can cause trouble. If Mars is placed in Cancer in opposition to its exaltation sign Capricorn, it also has no dignity (being in its 'fall') and will similarly work out in a negative way. All planets have signs in which they are very strong or very weak according to the list below.

Sun. Strong: in its own sign Leo, exalted in Aries. Weak: in detriment in Aquarius opposite Leo and in fall in Libra opposite Aries.

Moon. Strong: in its own sign Cancer and exalted in Taurus. Weak: in detriment in Capricorn and in fall in Scorpio.

Mercury. Strong: in its own signs Gemini and Virgo. Weak: in detriment in Sagittarius and in detriment and fall in Pisces. Virgo is Mercury's sign and exaltation, so it is extremely strong there.

Venus. Strong: in its own signs Taurus and Libra, in exaltation in Pisces. Weak: in detriment in Aries and Scorpio in fall in Virgo.

Mars. Strong: in its own signs Aries and Scorpio and exalted in Capricorn. Weak in detriment in Libra and Taurus and in fall in Cancer.

Jupiter. Strong in its own signs Sagittarius and Pisces and exalted in Cancer. Weak: in detriment in Gemini and Virgo, in fall in Capricorn.

Saturn. Strong in its own signs Aquarius and Capricorn and exalted in Libra. Weak: in detriment in Leo and Cancer, in fall in Aries

Only classical rulership applies here, so Jupiter rules Pisces, Mars rules Scorpio and Saturn rules Aquarius. The outer planets have no role in this pattern, which is rigidly logical and easy to remember. Some astrologers do not use the term 'in detriment', preferring 'exiled'. However detriment seems to describe better what this state means; the positive power a planet may have is absent, it is severely damaged. The normally positive working planet Jupiter for example is difficult when it is in detriment.

Placement in its own sign, exaltation, detriment and fall are the most important dignities, describing the main differences in planetary power. There are three other smaller positive dignities of which the elemental attribution is the most important. A planet which is placed in a sign of which the elemental nature accords well with its own nature, has some power, although definitely not so much as a planet in its own sign or exaltation. If a planet is placed in the right element it is called in triplicity in classical astrology. Triplicity is simply another word for element. It is easy to check whether a planet is placed in its triplicity. The first step is to check whether we have a day chart or a night chart. This is easy; if the Sun is above the horizon (in houses 7 to 12) it is daytime. If the Sun is below the horizon (in houses 1 to 6) it is night. If this is clear we apply the following rules:

Day Charts
Sun, Venus, Mars and Saturn may get extra power by placement in a suitable sign.

Essential dignity by triplicity: Sun in Fire signs, Saturn in Air signs, Mars in Water signs, Venus in Earth signs.

Night Charts
Jupiter, the Moon, Mars and Mercury may get extra power by placement in a suitable sign.

Essential dignity by triplicity: Jupiter in Fire signs, Mercury in Air signs, Mars in Water signs, the Moon in Earth signs.

There is also another system in which every element is allocated three planets instead of two. Some classical astrologers claim that this system mentioned by Dorotheus of Sidon is better because it is older. In practice this point cannot be proven and the two-ruler system is as ancient as the three-ruler system. In all branches of astrology the two-ruler system is effective and it can be used in medical astrology.

Besides triplicities there also the minor dignities term (termini: boundaries) and face (or decanate). These give a planet a small amount of extra power but not much. The terms are assessed on the basis of five planetary zones into which every sign can be divided, in each zone one planet is placed in its 'term'. Faces work in the same way but divide the signs into three zones of ten degrees each. These minor dignities give much less power than the other dignities but will sometimes be important. An overview of all the five dignities is given below.

SIGNS	HOUSES OF THE PLANETS	EXALTATION	TRIPLICITY OF PLANETS		THE TERMS OF THE PLANETS					THE FACES OF THE PLANETS			DETRIMENT	FALL
			Di.	Noc.										
♈	♂ D	☉ 19	☉	♃	♃ 6	♀ 14	☿ 21	♂ 26	♄ 30	♂ 10	☉ 20	♀ 30	♀	♄
♉	♀ N	☽ 3	♀	☽	♀ 8	☿ 15	♃ 22	♄ 20	♂ 30	☿ 10	☽ 20	♄ 30	♂	
♊	☿ D	☊ 3	♄	☿	☿ 7	♃ 14	♀ 21	♄ 25	♂ 30	♃ 10	♂ 20	☉ 30	♃	
♋	☽ N D	♃ 15	♂	♂	♂ 6	♃ 13	☿ 20	♀ 27	♄ 30	♀ 10	☿ 20	☽ 30	♄	♂
♌	☉ N D		☉	♃	♄ 6	☿ 13	♀ 19	♃ 25	♂ 30	♄ 10	♃ 20	♂ 30	♄	
♍	☿ N	☿ 15	♀	☽	☿ 7	♀ 13	♃ 18	♄ 24	♂ 30	☉ 10	♀ 20	☿ 30	♃	♀
♎	♀ D	♄ 21	♄	☿	♄ 6	♀ 11	♃ 19	☿ 24	♂ 30	☽ 10	♄ 20	♃ 30	♂	☉
♏	♂ N		♂	♂	♂ 6	♃ 14	♀ 21	☿ 27	♄ 30	♂ 10	☉ 20	♀ 30	♀	☽
♐	♃ D	☋ 3	☉	♃	♃ 8	♀ 14	☿ 19	♄ 25	♂ 30	☿ 10	☽ 20	♄ 30	☿	
♑	♄ N	♂ 28	♀	☽	♀ 6	☿ 12	♃ 19	♂ 25	♄ 30	♃ 10	♂ 20	☉ 30	☽	♃
♒	♄ D		♄	☿	♄ 6	☿ 12	♀ 20	♃ 25	♂ 30	♀ 10	☿ 20	☽ 30	☉	
♓	♃ N	♀ 27	♂	♂	♀ 8	♃ 14	☿ 20	♂ 26	♄ 30	♄ 10	♃ 20	♂ 30	♀	☿

Figure 2. Table of Essential Dignities

From left to right this table shows for each sign the planets that rule it and the planets which 'have dignity' there. The first column gives the signs, the second column the sign rulers and the third column the exaltation rulers. The figures in the exaltation column indicate the actual degree in the sign where the planet is said to be at its most exalted. The fourth column shows the triplicity, (first the ruler in a day chart, then the ruler in a night chart).

Columns 5 to 9 give the terms and columns 10 to 12 the faces. The face rulers have authority over ten-degree zones, which are also called decanates. The final two columns show the planets in their detriment and fall.

As an example, we can take Mercury in the ninth degree of Taurus in a diurnal chart. How much dignity does Mercury get there? The sign ruler of Taurus is Venus and the exaltation ruler is the Moon, so these planets have lots of power to work in a positive way there. Mercury will have no dignity through rulership or exaltation. The Lord of the Earth triplicity is Venus in this diurnal chart, so Mercury does not receive any essential dignity through triplicity either. But Mercury does have some dignity by term. The planet is placed in the second term of Taurus between 8 and 15 degrees and this is the term Mercury rules. He is in the right place by term. The first decanate of Taurus, the first ten-degree zone of the sign, is also ruled by Mercury, so he also gets some strength through face. We can then say that Mercury has term and face dignity, which is not much, but it is better than nothing and much better than debilitation by fall or detriment.

Another expression which must be explained is peregrine. A planet is peregrine when it has no dignity at all, positive or negative. It is not placed in its own sign or in exaltation, triplicity, term, face, detriment or fall. Peregrine means drifting; it is not bad, it is not good, it just has no direction. That is why it tends to be unhelpful though because things that have no direction can be seduced quite easily. It is often said that a planet is in detriment or fall *and* peregrine because it has no positive dignity, but this is incorrect; a planet in a bad state is clearly bad, whereas a drifting planet drifts and this not the same thing. It cannot be neutral and bad at the same time. It is important to think logically in astrology.

We also read a lot about benefics and malefics. The benefics are Jupiter and Venus and these planets tend to have a pleasant effect for us, but this is only true if they have some essential dignity; their benefic nature is diminished as they lose dignity. Jupiter in detriment in Virgo for example can no longer be called benefic; it is an 'accidental' malefic and will not work out well. Saturn and Mars are malefics by nature and tend to have unpleasant effects. However, if the malefics have essential dignity they lose much of their malefic character and may even work out well. The three remaining planets (Sun, Moon, Mercury) are more or less neutral in this respect although the same dignity principle applies; the more essential dignity they have the more positive their effects are.

Accidental dignity

The level of essential dignity or planetary power shows the planet's quality, or how purely it can be its own beneficial self. Venus in Libra is totally Venus and in this condition the planet can act according to its nature. The other kind of dignity called accidental shows something else: the force with which a planet can manifest in the world. The point is not whether this planet is working as it was meant according to its nature, but rather how strong is its influence in the world. Accidental dignity measures quantity, essential dignity measures quality. We can use the simple rules below to assess the degree of accidental dignity:

Strong: placement in an angular house, house 11, fast movement (not for Saturn), direct movement, no narrow aspects from malefics, joy (see below), conjunction with the favourable fixed stars Spica or Regulus.

Moderate: placement in houses 2, 3, 5 or 9.

Weak: conjunction or opposition with the Sun (combust), retrograding, placement in houses 6, 8 or 12, very slow movement (not for Saturn), narrow aspects with malefics, besiegement (placement between aspects with two malefics), in opposition with the house of its joys, on the malefic fixed star Algol.

The moon is weak when waning and strong when waxing. In the *via combusta*, the 'burnt road' (15 Libra to 15 Scorpio) the Moon is weakened too.

The North Node expands and strengthens and a conjunction with the North Node is generally positive. However when the cause of the illness is conjunct this expansive force it is not favourable. The South Node will diminish things and inhibit, and is mostly negative.

Joy is accidental dignity derived from a placement in a 'good' house, a house in which the planet feels at home by nature: Mercury in house 1, the Moon in house 3, Venus in house 5, Mars in house 6, the Sun in house 9, Jupiter in house 11 and Saturn in house 12. A planet in its joy feels good and therefore has more force to manifest itself in the world. A planet in opposition with its house of joy does not feel good and so is weakened.

A very damaging debilitation is combustion, a conjunction with the Sun. When the orb of conjunction is less than 8.30 degrees it is called combustion. If it is between 8.30 and 17.30 degrees it is termed 'under the Sun's beams', also difficult but not as malefic as real combustion. Combustion can also take place through an opposition to the Sun, with the same orb as when conjunct. When a planet is exactly conjunct the Sun it is called cazimi and this is extremely powerful. The orb for cazimi is 17.30 minutes of arc, so we do not often encounter this.

The phases of movement around a planet retrograding and becoming direct again are very important, especially with a view to prognosis. If a planet comes to a standstill – stationary – it is weak and vulnerable, but there is a noticeable difference between a planet turning to become direct after a period of retrogradation and a planet about to become retrograde for the first time. Turning direct is an indication of a strong improvement, and the patient will probably get better soon. Becoming retrograde however is a sign that things will get much worse.

Finally there are some powerful fixed stars which are important in medical horary astrology. Spica, at 23 Libra, is protective and points to a favourable outcome. Algol (26 Taurus) is extremely malefic just like Antares (9 Sagittarius), Alcyone (29 Taurus) and Vindemiatrix (10 Libra). Algol simply tells us that the outcome will be bad, Antares is a death star which ends cycles and Alcyone points to blindness and an unfavourable outcome. Vindemiatrix indicates an inflated ego and overestimation of one's powers, so is not very positive if the significator of the doctor or the treatment is placed on this star. Aldebaran at 9 Gemini finally points to much success and a new beginning.

The importance of the fixed stars depends on the nature of the medical question. In a question about an eye operation all stars which refer to blindness, for example nebulae, will have a negative meaning (see Appendix A). The system of accidental dignities may be refined further, but this is mostly important in natal astrology. For medical astrology which is mainly horary astrology, we do not need these refinements. In most cases we can clearly analyse a chart on the basis of the dignities mentioned above.

So, to clarify: suppose in the horary chart of a medical question the liver is important. The liver is given to house 5, and let us suppose its ruler is Saturn which is placed in Leo on the descendant, about to become retrograde. The system of essential dignities tells us that Saturn is in detriment, which indicates that the liver is in a bad state. Because Saturn is on the descendant, in opposition with the ascendant (the body), this has much influence on health. It is to be expected that the condition of the liver will worsen because Saturn will turn retrograde. In this way the condition of organs and the strength of negative or positive influences can be evaluated.

Receptions

Receptions are of crucial importance in astrology. They show what effects planets have on each other and whether they damage or help each other. To assess these connections we need the table of essential dignities. An example will show how this works. Suppose a client has a question about a disease and Mercury in Aries turns out to be the cause of the disease. The most important receptions Mercury makes from Aries will guide the analysis of the chart and show the effects the illness has on the body.

The general rule in analysing receptions is that a planet in a sign will have a positive effect on its dispositors and a negative effect on the planets which have their fall and detriment in this sign. So Mercury in Aries has a negative influence on Venus (which is in detriment in Aries) and Saturn (which has its fall in Aries). It works positively on Mars (the sign ruler of Aries) and the Sun (which has its exaltation in Aries). As we are interested in medical charts and cause of diseases in this book, the negative receptions are the most important. These receptions show in which parts of the body the illness will manifest; but if we ask the question as to whether a treatment or operation would do any good, positive receptions may also be important because they show in which body parts the treatment or operation will have a favourable effect.

Through the network of receptions we can map all these connections between the relevant significators systematically; something which is always important and often crucial and we should always carry out such an analysis. In most cases we can limit ourselves to the most powerful receptions such as fall, detriment, sign rulership and exaltation. Sometimes a reception through triplicity rulership will show something important but receptions through the minor dignities of term and face are seldom of essential importance in medical horary astrology.

Planet and humor

Not only the signs but also the planets can be characterized by the humors. This is the final theoretical building-block we need for the practical work of diagnosis. The division of the planets on the basis of the humors is related to the combined play of signs and planets which is the essence of astrology. The signs describe the general potencies, the possibilities the cosmos offers. The planets are the dynamic factors of formation which give the potencies a real form on earth.

In a sense planets are formed from the same materials as signs but they represent these elemental energies in a more concrete, active and specific form. As we saw in astrological anatomy, the planets are energy streams in the body, which take on form in the functions of several organs. They are of the following humoral nature.

The Fire planets Sun and Mars are hot and dry
The Water planets Moon and Venus are cold and moist
The Earth planets Saturn and Mercury are cold and dry
The Air planet Jupiter is hot and moist

Because medical astrology is based on the contrast between hot and cold and dry and moist, the nature of the planet is crucial in diagnosis. There are differences in strength: Saturn is colder and drier than Mercury, the Moon is colder and moister than Venus, Mars is hotter and drier than the Sun.

The only thing which may seem a bit strange in this theory is the cold and dry nature of flexible, active Mercury. There is however a reason for this. The planet is dry because it does not really connect; a real connection is described by moisture. Mercury moves quickly and consequently his connections are only of a fleeting nature. Mercury is also cold – he does not add energy like Mars for example. He only has a conductive function; he creates a connection but it is no more than that. Now we have all the basic knowledge we need to be able to make the diagnosis.

Method of diagnosis

Let us see what actually happens if a medical horary question is asked. The client will describe his problem through email, telephone or in a letter. It is of course not important in which way the question reaches the astrologer; the moment the question is understood by the astrologer, it is 'born', and then we can calculate a chart.

And what is the essential point in most medical questions? The client usually wants to know what is wrong with his body, what is it that is doing him harm and making him ill? The body in question is the most important factor in the chart and this is the ruler of the first house, Lord 1. Although you hear so often that we must analyse the sixth house of illness, Lord 6 has no role in medical questions. The reason for this is the very nature of horary astrology. The chart of the question about the diseased body will show exactly that, the diseased body and the forces and developments harming it. The horary chart shows the illness in its entirety, so we do not need a special house to indicate disease. The great advantage of horary astrology is that it is totally specific for the querent's situation.

There are two kinds of charts in which Lord 6 does play a role, but they are very different. Firstly there is the natal chart which describes all aspects of life. In natal charts the sixth house and its ruler do show the individual disease tendencies, something which will be further discussed in Chapter 12. This knowledge can be used to advise on preventive measures. The crucial difference with horary charts is that the natal chart covers life in its entirety, of which illness is only a part. We cannot simply take the ruler of the first house as the diseased body in the natal chart because the natal chart is not a chart for a medical question.

Secondly, there is the decumbiture chart in which the sixth house is certainly important. The Latin verb *decumbere* means to lie down. This kind of chart is calculated for the moment the client is overwhelmed by the disease and has to lie down in bed. It is simply the start of the disease, its 'birth'. This chart is an event chart, with no question being asked about the specific situation. Therefore we do look at Lord 6 which may for example be in opposition with the Moon, the Sun or Lord 1 at that moment of lying down. This may give important information in making a diagnosis.

It is crucial to distinguish clearly between horary charts and decumbitures as they are analysed quite differently. Many classical authorities, and even the great master of horary, William Lilly, mixed up the two charts and the result is enormous confusion. Example charts in the old texts are in most cases decumbitures, and the methods used for analysing decumbitures are not suitable for horaries. The emphasis on decumbitures in the traditional texts has to do with the way medical astrologers practised their profession in those days. On the basis of the decumbiture chart a so-called 'figure of sixteen houses' can be calculated. In this figure the doctor/astrologer could see when to apply certain healing measures and when the crisis was to be expected. The medical astrologer in current times does not treat his patients in this way any more; the majority of cases in those days was acute, and such cases would now be treated by modern doctors. Neither are there many clients who can tell their time of lying down because they do not note this and there will not always be such a moment. Decumbitures have become unimportant because the nature of the astromedical consultation has changed, (although the whole method and the figure of the sixteen houses could still be used in principle).

The figure of the sixteen houses is calculated on the basis of the movement of the Moon. Charts are drawn up for the moments the Moon is in square, opposition and again conjunct its initial decumbiture position. This gives the framework for the development of the disease. If the opposition chart is positive it indicates recovery after two weeks and this would be the moment to apply the most powerful healing measures. The astrologer would always work along with the natural flow of the disease. Apart from the 90 degree chart (valid for a week) we also have 45 degree charts (half a week) and a 22.30 degree chart (less than two days). These additional charts give extra information about the development of the disease; as when moments of great heat might be indicated (Mars on the ascendant for example) or when extra cooling measures would be appropriate. The figure is only for timing and fine tuning treatment; the decumbiture is used for drawing up the diagnosis and the treatment plan.

Something else worth mentioning is that we might read about charts being calculated for the moment the urine of the diseased person was brought by a servant or a member of the family. Doctors used to analyse the colour of the urine to provide information about the humor causing the problem. If the urine was reddish we could suspect a yellow choler or fire excess. When the servant arrived at the house of the astrologer-doctor with his bottle of urine this was implicitly a question from his master: "What is wrong with me?" So the chart for the moment the urine was brought could also be treated as a horary, and has to be distinguished sharply from a decumbiture.

Analysis
These days we do not have to worry about decumbitures and charts with "urine brought by servants" any more. Classical medical astrologers today work almost exclusively with medical horaries and bottles of urine are no longer brought to our door-steps. In most cases the analysis of a medical horary is quite simple, although there will always be the more complicated and challenging examples. We can use the following

approach. Firstly we determine which planet is Lord 1 in the horary chart. This is the querent's diseased body. Then we compare the humoral nature of this planet with the humoral nature of the sign in which it is placed. If the body is Mercury in Aries, we have a cold and dry planet – Mercury – placed in a hot and dry sign.

If the humoral nature of Lord 1 differs from the humoral nature of the sign, Lord 1 is in an environment in which he does not feel at ease. That is the reason he is dis-eased. Because signs are only the backgrounds to the planets, we look at the dispositor of the sign in which Lord 1 is placed. This planet is the cause of the disease; as Lord 1's dispositor it has a lot of power over the body. So if Mercury in Aries is Lord 1, the sign position of Mars gives us the cause of the disease.

Suppose Mercury's dispositor Mars is placed in the sign of Cancer, then we have Mars in Cancer as the cause of the disease: the position of a planet in a sign describes the illness. The next general rule is that the nature of the sign in which Lord 1's dispositor is placed indicates which humor or element is present in the body in excess. Mars in the Water sign of Cancer identifies the Water element as the root of the problem: excess phlegm is the disease cause.

Of course, the planet is also important. The sign is the background, the deeper level, but this does influence the planet. In the case of Mars in Cancer this means that the excess phlegm from Cancer has disturbed the martial energy stream. This unbalanced Mars is part of the problem, part of the disease pattern. It may manifest in certain fiery symptoms, for example in the skin, but these symptoms do not mean it is a Fire disease.

A book which is of great value in making diagnosis sharper is Richard Saunders' *The Astrological Judgement and Practice of Physick* which was published in 1677. This book is a real treasure chest of medical knowledge and very effective in practice. *The Astrological Judgement and Practice of Physick* is divided into three parts. The first part is general, treating of traditional medicine and classical medical astrology. The second part is practical and very valuable in making a diagnosis as Saunders gives a description of the pattern of symptoms for all planetary positions. We can find a description of Mars in Cancer in the chapter on Mars' diseases, and Saunders says that the main cause is excess phlegm or water coming from the watery sign of Cancer. As a second additional cause he mentions fire or yellow choler coming from the Fire planet Mars. The illness may manifest as an inflammatory symptom, but the deeper cause is the phlegm excess.

Having found the cause in Saunders' lists, we can look up the remedy in the third part of the book. Saunders gives a list of remedies for all planetary positions, mostly single herbs or mixtures of herbs. Sometimes these are complicated traditional recipes which were prepared by apothecaries in those days and which could be purchased from them. As there are no traditional apothecaries any more and preparation of these recipes is often difficult, we can no longer use many of these treatments, but often simpler means are mentioned which turn out to be most successful in practice.

For the planetary positions Saunders does not only give the cause in terms of humoral excess, he also mentions how severe the problem is. This is traditionally given as one of four degrees of severity. The first degree is a light disturbance, the second and third degrees are real problems and a fourth degree illness can often not be healed or may indeed prove fatal. The degree of humoral disturbance increases as the year gets older. So a planet in Aries points towards a light yellow choler excess, whereas the same planet in Leo shows a much more severe problem and a position in Sagittarius gives a fatal illness or one that is very difficult to heal. The same idea applies to the other three humors, so Pisces gives much more phlegm than Cancer. On the basis of the horary chart, possibly combined with Saunders' book, we can make a reliable diagnosis and advise on effective treatment.

Practical example: arthritis

A practical example will clarify how theoretical knowledge can be applied in practice. A client had been suffering from arthritis for some time, and wanted to know what he could do about it. The arthritis manifested in one of his toes causing great difficulty in walking during the bouts. The client's doctor had prescribed pain-killers and anti-inflammatory remedies. This was effective against the symptoms but the problem kept coming back. The chart of the question is analysed rigidly according to fixed rules. The querent's body is the first house ruler – in this case Venus, ruler of the Libra ascendant. Venus is a cold and moist planet but it is placed in a hot and dry sign, Leo. This is the cause of the dis-ease.

To see what this means we go to the sign ruler of Leo, the Sun. The Sun is placed in Virgo and this combination of planet-in-sign is the cause of the arthritis.

The Sun in Virgo indicates an excess of black choler, Virgo is an Earth sign. This melancholic excess has disturbed the function of the Sun as a planetary energy. Mixed with the black choler we find some yellow choler coming from the hot and dry Sun. The Sun is not the deepest cause of the disease – this is the melancholy excess – but it is part of the illness. Saunders says that this placement indicates cold of the second degree and dryness of the third degree. The problem is considerable but it can be healed. Furthermore he writes that it causes stiffness of the sinews. This is not exactly right but stiffness because of cold or dryness is the picture of the disease.

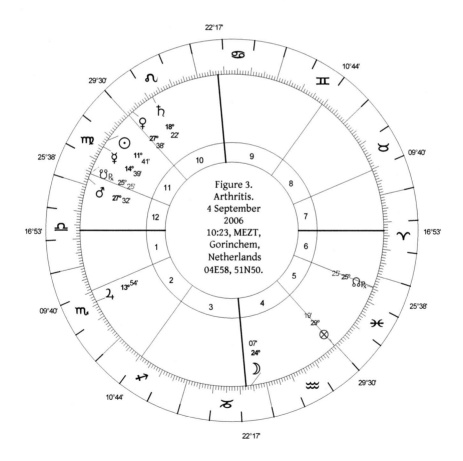

Figure 3.
Arthritis.
4 September 2006
10:23, MEZT,
Gorinchem,
Netherlands
04E58, 51N50.

On the basis of this description we can imagine what is going on here; we easily get a clear-cut image. There is much dryness, so there is hardly any moisture in the joints. Moisture is needed to lubricate things, as without moisture we will have friction. Dry surfaces rasp and scratch over each other and this gives heat. This is exactly the image the chart shows: cold and dry black choler is the deepest cause and this results in friction and heat, the inflammatory symptom. So what should be treated is the deepest cause and preferably also the secondary cause, the unbalanced hot and dry solar energy. Part 3 of this book describes methods of treatment, so this will not be discussed here.

In the chart we can see some clear illustrations of techniques which have been described in the previous chapters. It is noticeable that Mars is on the twelfth house cusp and planets on cusps relevant to the situation often give important information. Anatomically the twelfth house refers to the feet and indeed the problem manifested in one of the toes. Fiery Mars also shows the inflammatory symptom again. But it is crucial to understand that it is only a result of a deeper imbalance in the whole system: a black choler excess.

The Sun in Virgo is also clearly involved with Mercury which is close by. Mercury is combust but the Sun is also in the sign of Mercury. The planet does not give the cause of the disease but it is connected to it in a way. Mercury rules the twelfth house, symbolizing the feet, another indication that there is a foot problem. You can also analyse the effectiveness and power of the treatment that is given, indicated by the tenth house and its Lord. This is the treatment that is being given, NOT the treatment that should be given. In this chart the Moon is in Capricorn where it is very weak in its detriment, showing that the Moon has hardly any power to do anything really good, so the arthritis kept coming back. The cold and dry nature of the remedy is shown by Lord 1's placement in the cold and dry sign of Capricorn.

Painkillers and anti-inflammatory medication have a cooling and drying effect so the treatment added more dryness and cold to a body which was already too dry and cold. The inflammatory symptom will disappear but it will also increase the imbalance which is the deepest cause of the disease. The treatment maintains the illness and this is something we see more and more often when medication is prescribed. Every time the symptom reappears it is suppressed, but the medication makes the body increasingly colder and drier. Finally, the black choler excess will manifest as a more serious disease.

The traditional treatment was successful in this case, and the arthritis did not come back.

Sometimes it may be necessary to remove the symptom first. In this case we would want to subdue the painful inflammation but there are many effective natural measures which may achieve that, sometimes applied externally and locally without disturbing the body further. The most elegant means are crystals, which will be discussed further in Chapter 9. An arthritis attack for example may be treated by placing a chrysopras or a garnet (a grossular) on the skin, and the pain and the inflammatory symptoms will decrease rapidly.

If we know the deeper cause of the disease a whole battery of measures can be applied to treat the disease on the physical, psychological and spiritual levels. The treatment plan covers dietary measures, herbal teas, spagyric or alchemical essences, herbal tinctures, crystals, life style changes, psychology and spiritual factors, which have contributed to the development of the disease. This will all be discussed extensively in Part 3 of this book.

Yellow choler and thyroid gland

Although black choler is the most damaging humor, the other three humors can also cause problems. In this example the trouble is not black choler, but yellow choler. The question is what could be done about an acute osteoporosis which had recently developed. The doctors decided they wanted to perform an operation to remove the thyroid gland which had become overactive and was causing the accelerated osteoporosis.

Again the chart very clearly shows the whole medical situation. We will follow the usual standard method for analysing medical horaries. The ruler of the first house is Mars, the significator of the body. Mars is a hot and dry planet placed in the cold and dry sign of Virgo. So the client is dis-eased because of this placement and its dispositor will indicate the cause of the disease; in other words, its dispositor with its sign placement is the disease. This is Mercury in the hot, dry sign of Leo. So it is the hot and dry yellow choler that has caused the disease, an excess of Fire.

Fire accelerates the processes in the body, and in this case it is the thyroid gland that is overactive, which very much fits the idea of too much yellow choler. It is striking that Mercury has just entered the hot and dry sign of Leo and the illness has developed only recently. Also the conjunction of the Sun and Saturn near the MC cannot be overlooked. Saturn is the general significator of the bones and is very important here.

Planets which harm the bones may provide additional information about the disease situation. This leads us back to Mercury in Leo placed in the sign in which Saturn is in its detriment, we then say that Mercury receives Saturn in its detriment. The practical effect is that any planet in Leo will harm Saturn. This is how we use negative reception: a planet in a sign harms the planets which are in detriment and fall in this sign. It is clear that the cause of the illness, Mercury, in Leo, harms Saturn: the bones.

The dominating Sun on the MC also has a role to play. It is conjunct Saturn, which is combust, and the Sun receives Saturn into detriment, which is negative for Saturn. The Sun has a detrimental influence on the condition of the bones. The Sun is the Lord of the tenth house which describes the medication or treatment given, so the medication is not working.

The solution is to put out the Fire that has caused the whole problem. Cooling and moisturizing foods and herbs which lead Fire out of the body are the right measures. The symptom of acute hyperactivity of the thyroid gland can be treated with a rock-crystal or rhinestone necklace worn close to the skin. The patient should if possible stop taking medication. The chart also shows that an operation is not a good idea as it will only make things worse. In Chapter 10 we discuss how to deal with these questions about treatments and operations.

Special cases

Most medical horaries can be analysed following the method outlined above and in this way we can give an effective advice on treatment. However there are special cases in which the standard method will not work. There are two categories: placement of Lord 1 in a sign corresponding to his humoral nature, and placement of Lord 1 in the sign he rules himself. An example of the first category of a planet in a sign corresponding to its humoral nature is Mercury in Capricorn. This is a cold and dry planet in a cold and dry sign. The reason that the body has become unbalanced is not necessarily given by Capricorn's ruler Saturn.

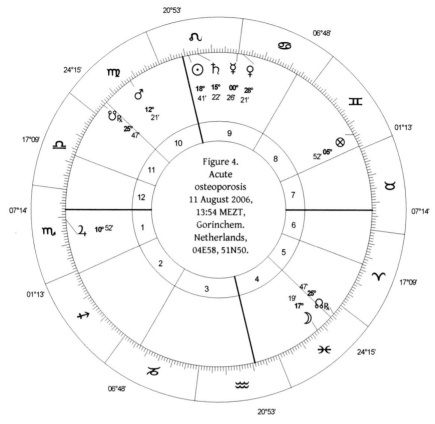

Figure 4.
Acute
osteoporosis
11 August 2006,
13:54 MEZT,
Gorinchem.
Netherlands,
04E58, 51N50.

In such a case the chart has to be searched further for planets harming the body, indicated by Lord 1 in the chart.

Possible causes are: a planet separating from a harmful aspect with Lord 1; a planet in negative reception with Lord 1; a planet from which the Moon is separating; an elevated planet high in the chart; an angular planet, or even Lord 1's dispositor (especially when it is essentially debilitated) or Lord 1 itself (especially when it is retrograding). Also the Sun may be the disease cause as if Lord 1 is combust, the Sun harms the body. Sometimes you have to search the chart for a while but almost always the cause will be identified in this way. This will be clear because for example a planet may harm Lord 1 through negative reception while the Moon is separating from this same planet in the chart. It is as if the chart is pointing out the problem. Maybe this sounds a little complicated, but in practice these additional techniques will give you a clear indication of the cause of the disease.

The second category of special cases to which the standard method cannot be applied concerns Lord 1 in its own sign, as for example Venus in Libra. It is then its own dispositor and indeed Lord 1 itself may be the cause of the disease. But just as in the previous chart, we need to check for other likely culprits in the form of damaging aspects, recent Moon aspects, negative reception and combustion. If there are no indications to be found that another planet is the cause of the disease, the planet which is Lord 1 will be the body and the disease. This is all the more probable if it is retrograding or if the sign is different from Lord 1 humorally, for example hot dry Mars in wet cold Scorpio.

It is clear here that the Moon is only of secondary importance in medical horaries. The Moon shows the querent's emotional focus and not what is wrong with his body and therefore Lord 1 is the most important factor. However the most recent Moon aspect may give additional information about a symptom or something else which plays a role in the whole disease process. The Moon will not show the real deeper cause on its own. Medical horaries are different from 'normal' horary charts, in which the Moon counts as a full co-significator for the querent.

An example of a complex question in which the standard method could not be applied is the following query about the possible treatment of MS (multiple sclerosis). This case was diagnosed as MS but in traditional medicine it is different because it thinks of diagnoses in terms of humoral excess. Lord 1 is Mercury retrograding in Virgo. This gives a clear image of the disease: Mercury significator of the nervous system does not function well, because it is retrograde. It is also in Virgo, a very cold and dry sign. Lord 1 is however in a sign it rules and with which it is humorally compatible.

We have to look for another cause. Nearby is the Sun, so Mercury is damaged by combustion and the Sun could be the disease. But because combustion takes place in the sign Mercury rules this combustion cannot be seen as very damaging, it is more like a mutual reception. This is because Mercury as the sign and exaltation ruler of Virgo has a lot of power over the Sun and this will decrease the negative effect of combustion considerably. So the Sun cannot be the disease cause as it has not such a negative influence on Mercury. The disease is Mercury in Virgo itself, for there is no other acceptable cause to be found in the chart. A nervous system which is debilitated by too much cold and dryness also gives a rather precise image of what is going on in the case of MS.

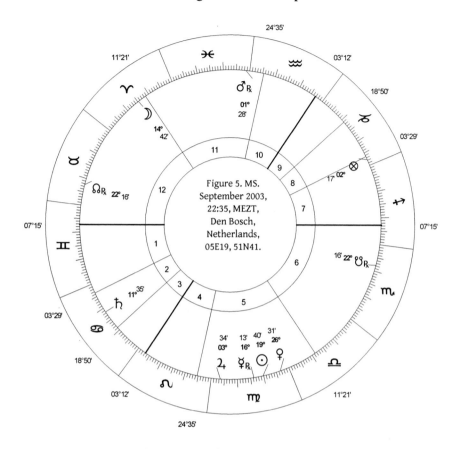

Figure 5. MS.
September 2003,
22:35, MEZT,
Den Bosch,
Netherlands,
05E19, 51N41.

An exceptional category of charts comprises those which cannot be analysed by applying a method, standard or non-standard. In astrology not everything can be defined through rigid rules, the cosmos is not a mechanical computer, it is a living organism. Even though we said earlier that astrology is completely logical, logical and mechanical (machinelike) are different things. Logic means being understood on the basis of principles.

A good example of 'organic' logic is a planet that has just passed the sign boundary. If such a planet is the cause of the disease and the question is about a chronic problem, the position of the planet in the new sign cannot possibly be the cause. The chronic problem will have been there for some time so the cause is given by the planet's position in the previous sign, the one it has just left. Always remain flexible and check if the chart mirrors the situation.

5

An Imbalance of Energy

Prognosis

The diagnosis and the treatment advice based on the horary are usually the most important parts of the medical interpretation of the chart, but this is not always so. Sometimes prognosis is the crucial point. A special case in my practice was a client suffering from Crohn's disease, a serious chronic inflammation of the large intestines. The doctor suggested an operation, but the querent had her doubts and asked how her condition would develop in the next few months. Would an operation really be necessary?

The querent in the chart is a retrograde Mercury – not very surprising because the client is seriously ill and retrogradation is a serious affliction. But Mercury is losing speed, it will soon be direct again and it is leaving combustion. This shows that an enormous improvement of her condition is to be expected. So it would be sensible to wait – if possible – and see if this improvement would indeed come. Within three months the querent had recovered completely without the need for an operation.

In this chart prognosis is the main thing and the movement of Lord 1/the body through the chart is one of the most important factors on which we can base a reliable prognosis. It is crucial however that the chart gives the prognosis as a continuation of the given situation! Suppose someone is suffering from migraine and Lord 1 is going to aspect the cause of the disease, the condition of the patient will worsen – but only if no measures are taken.

The chart shows the situation as it is and how it could develop if nothing is done. Of course this is not so if the question is explicitly about the effects of an operation or treatment. In that case the chart shows what will happen if we decide to undergo the operation and/or treatment. In fact this question would be: if I do this what will happen next? As always in horary astrology the precise understanding of the context in which the question is asked is crucial for a correct interpretation of the chart. If you understand the question clearly, you have done half the interpretation.

If the question is about an illness, the development of the illness can be predicted from the movement of Lord 1 and some other factors. It is not a positive sign if Lord 1 is about to aspect the cause of the disease or a planet which may harm it. Neither is it good if Lord 1 is about to enter the sign of its detriment or fall, this indicates a worsening like increasing combustion by the Sun or turning retrograde. Another factor of great importance in prognosis is the nature of the sign in which the cause of the disease is placed. A cardinal sign points to a disease which will develop fast, a mutable sign to a problem that comes and goes and a fixed sign a deep-seated, fixed illness. It refers to the mode of manifestation.

However, it is also important to find out how deeply the humoral balance has been disturbed. In Saunders' book the degrees of disturbance can also be checked for every planetary position. This varies from lighter disturbances of the first degree in the beginning of the zodiac to heavy sometimes incurable disturbances in the late signs. The context of the disease is important in using these degrees as always in horary astrology. If a patient suffers from a chronic disease like MS, the third degree is indeed a very serious problem. But if we are talking about a headache of the fourth degree this indicates a serious headache, not a fatal one.

This knowledge can be used in a very precise way and the question about the acute osteoporosis in the last chapter (see page 47) is a good example. The cause of the illness is Mercury in Leo, a fixed sign which is not good because the problem is also fixed so will take some time to heal. Saunders gives for this position first degree dryness and second degree heat. This is encouraging, as although the illness is fixed the disturbance of the balance is not serious, relatively mild herbs and other mild measures may improve the condition. Mars as Lord 1 in the chart is not going to make any damaging aspects, so this is also positive.

The only thing which looks bad is that the cause of the disease is on its way to a square with Lord 2, the significator of the thyroid gland, the organ which is hyperactive because of the excess of heat and dryness in the system. Lord 2 signifies the thyroid gland because the gland is found in the throat and Lord 2 describes its condition. If the organ which is part of the problem comes into direct contact with the deeper cause, this cannot possibly mean anything positive, so we have to take measures to save the thyroid gland as soon as possible. These are based on the astrological analysis and can involve laying rock-crystals on the throat and drinking cooling and moistening teas.

Timing

The timing is given by the number of zodiac degrees Mercury still has to travel before the square is really made, in this case about twelve degrees. So we can expect a worsening of the thyroid gland's condition after twelve weeks or three months. A falling house like the ninth indicates a short time unit, a fixed sign a long time unit, so we should use a time unit per degree which is neither too long not too short. With a view to the nature of the disease and the developments, a day per degree would be too short and a month too long, so a week is the most logical choice.

This is the general method by which we can analyse the development of a disease. We look at the planet (in most cases Lord 1) which is on its way to – for example – a damaging aspect, a sign boundary or combustion. The number of degrees the significator still has to cover until it reaches this place is found in the ephemeris, a degree is taken as one time unit. However, it is not clear yet whether these units/degrees are hours, days, weeks, months or years. To determine this, the position of our significator (the applying planet) has be evaluated further.

The first factor is the sign it is in: a fixed sign is a long period of time, a mutable sign is in the middle and a cardinal sign is short. The second factor is house placement, an angular house in medical astrology almost always indicates a longer period of time, a succedent house is in the middle and a cadent house short. In this way we get two indications of which only long-long and short-short are not 'in the middle'. So it is more probable that we get a middle unit and in most cases it is clear from the context which time unit this is.

This method has been proven to work in practice, and means that the term 'cardinal house' which is often used for angular houses nowadays is wrong. Angular houses correspond to the fixed signs which both point to long time units. Angular houses are fixed because they are houses of manifestation in slow earthly reality. The fixed mode is the mode of manifestation in matter. The cardinal mode shows the fast-moving first impulse which precedes manifestation and the mutable mode refers to the succedent houses which follow on from manifestation and in which things return to their origin. So falling houses correspond to the fast-moving cardinal mode and succedent house to the middle units of the mutable mode.

In non-medical horaries this method has to be adapted sometimes, because a factor in an angular house is able to act. If the chart shows that this planet wants to act by receptions, then, and only then, an angular house indicates a short time unit. In medical horaries this is mostly irrelevant because disease processes cannot be influenced so easily by just wanting to act and having intention; the disease has its own rhythm of development. In medical horary astrology we can safely assume that angular houses refer to long time units.

So to draw up a good prognosis several factors have to taken into account, among which the movement of Lord 1 - the body - is the most important of all. If the condition of Lord 1 is going to worsen through an aspect with a malefic, by entering combustion, going retrograde or entering the sign of its fall or detriment, this is a very negative sign. Apart from the movement of Lord 1, the nature of the sign in which the significator of the illness is found (mutable, cardinal or fixed) and the degree of the humoral disturbance are also factors to be taken into account. Below two example charts are discussed to show how this can work in practice.

Case: psoriasis

This client has been suffering from psoriasis for a long time and the disease was getting worse again, which is why the question was asked. Following our standard method we look at the position of Lord 1, in this chart it is Mercury in the sign of Scorpio. Mercury is a cold and dry planet in a cold and moist Water sign, so the planet does not feel good here. This means that Mercury's dispositor will give the cause of the disease. This is Mars the ruler of Scorpio, itself also placed in this fixed Water sign, so the fixed waters of Scorpio are the deeper cause of the disease.

In his famous book, Saunders describes the diagnosis for this planetary position as cold and moist of the second degree: "...causing

Diseases of thick stinking Flegm and Water with red Choler, Flegm predominating..." This refers to the fixed phlegm stuck in the body because the sign always gives the main cause of the disease; the red choler comes from the very hot and dry planet Mars. Furthermore he says it leads to the "Small Pox in young and old", an apt description as the old medical terms were used in a much more global way than we are used to now. Small Pox (small pocks) would not only refer to the specific disease but to many ailments with fiery symptoms in the skin.

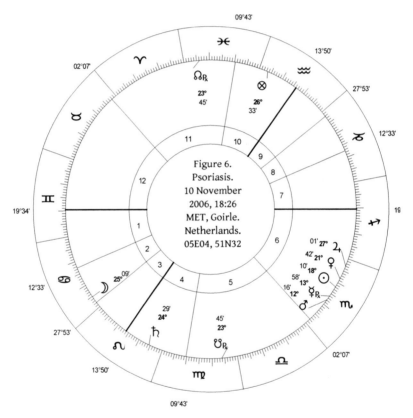

Figure 6. Psoriasis. 10 November 2006, 18:26 MET, Goirle. Netherlands. 05E04, 51N32

It is inspiring to realise that a horary chart of a medical question together with a book from 1677 can give the right diagnosis. Traditional medicine is still valid in all its aspects and has only been pushed aside by the rationalistic attitude of our modern culture. A horary chart always mirrors the situation concerning the question asked and this is very clear in this example. The reason for the question was that the illness was gradually worsening and we see that Lord 1 – the body – has just left a conjunction with the Sun and is on its way to Mars, the cause. This does not look good; the body which is in a bad condition – retrograding and combust – will soon contact the cause of the disease. This position between two damaging planets is called besiegement.

As the skin is clearly part of the problem here, it is a good idea to look at the condition of the general significator of the skin, Saturn. This planet is in a very bad condition indeed, in its detriment in hot and dry Leo. Not too long ago the cause of the disease made an opposition with the so-called antiscion of Saturn which is placed in the sixth degree of Taurus. Antiscia are mirror-points calculated by mirroring the planetary positions through an axis drawn from zero degrees Cancer to Capricorn. In horary charts, conjunctions and oppositions to antiscia must always be taken into account. In this chart we see that the cause of the disease made a contact with the skin through antiscion, which describes the situation well enough.

All significators are placed in fixed signs showing that it is a deep-rooted problem, which had been going on for some time. It is however positive that Saunders gives the diagnosis for this planetary position as a second-degree disturbance, a relatively mild illness that is certainly not incurable. In this way we can give a prognosis and can see in the chart what has happened before the question was asked by looking at the movements of the relevant significators. The dietary measures and the herbal teas which were prescribed on the basis of the chart were effective; soon the psoriasis started to recede and the vitality noticeably improved.

This case shows how essential a chart is. The deepest cause of the disease was moisture and cold, quite surprising for an illness with fiery and dry symptoms. You would think that excess Fire was the cause. But this is not the deepest cause although it is clearly part of the whole picture; hot and dry Mars is the planet which also describes the illness. It is this Mars which leads to the fiery symptoms, but the deeper reason for the imbalanced condition remains the cold and moist sign background, the fixed waters of Scorpio. The treatment should mainly aim at removing this excess phlegm.

It is illustrative to consider the meaning of Mars in Scorpio; what does the image tell us? What does it mean that this position is the disease?

The chart shows that the assertive fighting power of Mars does not function well because of the excess water in the system. It is as if we see a warrior under water. Remove the water and he will be able to fight again. The planetary picture could also be seen in the patient's behaviour: strongly assertive martial energy waves which change into phlegmatic exhaustion and sleeplessness. It takes lots of energy to fight under water. These phenomena all point to an unbalanced martial force which can not function in the right way because of the excess of Water.

It shows that the astrological symbolism is very broad; the imbalanced martial energy describes the ailment on many different layers of the organism. It does not only refer to the physical level, the psychological condition is part of it. The physical and the psychological are closely connected, seamlessly flowing over into each other and influencing each other. Too much phlegm may also be caused by grief, unshed tears and frustrating experiences, and in combination with the wrong dietary pattern this may lead to an illness like the one described here.

So food, herbs and life style have a strong influence on the psyche, and the psyche does influence the humoral balance. There is no isolated separate psyche and in the strict sense of the word no psychiatric or psychological illnesses. There are disturbances of the humoral balance which manifest most clearly on the psychological level, but these diseases can be healed in the same way as the more physical diseases by means of dietary changes, herbs, crystals and alchemical essences. I know of a case in which potatoes were effective in preventing recurring psychosis.

A last thing that strikes the eye in this chart is the fact that Mars is strong in its own sign. Unfortunately, this has no positive meaning because the chart points to this planetary position as the cause of the disease, and essential dignity does not count in this diagnosis. In our medical context the main things are heat/cold and dryness/moisture; even a very strong benefic like Jupiter in Pisces may lead to a serious phlegmatic disease because Pisces indicates an excess of phlegm. In medical astrology, dignity is mainly used to evaluate the condition of organs – when we have Lord 5 in fall, the liver is not in the best of conditions. It also plays a role in drawing up a treatment plan as we shall see later.

Case: 'Iliac Passion'

This client suffers from a digestive problem and could not keep much food in his stomach, as a consequence of which he had lost much weight. In this chart Lord 1 is Mars, a hot and dry planet placed in the hot and moist sign of Libra. Lord 1's nature does not fit that of the sign, so Venus in Libra – Mars' dispositor – is the cause of the illness. Saunders gives for Venus in Libra among other things "Cholick" and "pains and gripings in the belly". He describes the symptoms further as "...a Wind running up and down the body that is sometimes in the bowels and sometimes in the stomach and sometimes under the short ribs in the left side, with great pain..." This is called the 'Iliac Passion' an obstruction of the digestive tract which leads to vomiting. Again we have an apt description in this centuries-old book in which the real sources are much older than 1677.

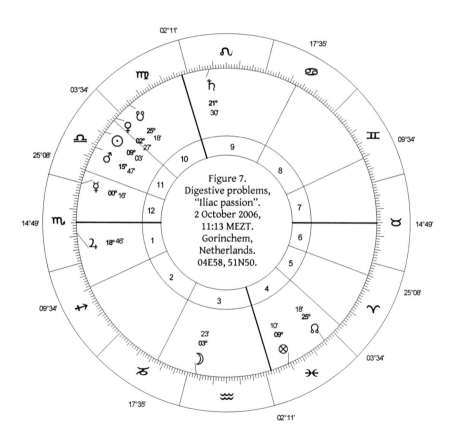

Figure 7.
Digestive problems,
"Iliac passion".
2 October 2006,
11:13 MEZT.
Gorinchem,
Netherlands.
04E58, 51N50.

Venus is placed in the sanguine air sign Libra, so too much blood is the deepest cause of the problem. Too much blood means not enough of the opposite humor, so Earth or black choler is lacking. Black choler keeps the food we eat in the body long enough to be digested, but in this case the excess Air forces the ingested food through the digestive tract too fast, leading to vomiting or "gripings in the belly". It moves in every direction, so the patient is not able to effectively digest his food.

A planet placed exactly on a cusp always deserves some attention, and here we have Venus very near cusp 11 in opposition with the fifth house cusp, the liver. Venus is also placed in the sign where Mars has its detriment; it receives Mars in detriment, so it damages the liver. Mars rules the fifth house and is in extremely bad condition, so the bad condition of the liver is surely of importance and we have to prescribe measures which improve the liver function. The houses the relevant significators rule can provide more information about factors which play a role in the cause of the illness. In this chart Venus is Lord 7 which may point to the possible involvement of relationship issues.

The prognosis does not look good. The Sun is applying to Mars – Lord 1, the body – an increasing combustion. This is one of the strongest afflictions possible and is a very negative sign that the combustion can only become stronger. We have to interfere as soon as possible because Lord 1 is also applying to a sextile with Saturn in detriment which looks unpleasant too. The measures we can take to get rid of the excess blood or Air are described in Part 3 of this book.

6

Cosmic Principles:
Sympathy and Antipathy

Evaporating and extinguishing

The method as discussed in Part 2 will give us a reliable diagnosis. A typical diagnosis would look like this: excess fixed phlegm of the second degree as a result of which the Mars function in the body has become unbalanced – as was the case in the psoriasis question. Treatment will be directed at restoring the humoral balance as the excess of moisture and cold has to be removed. By inserting more heat and dryness into the system the moisture and cold will be evaporated. It can be compared to morning mists lifting in the first warmth of the sun.

This is the simple principle of antipathy, fighting the cause of the problem with remedies of a contrary nature. If there is too much Fire, you can extinguish this by throwing Water on it. Water can be brought into the body in many ways, for example by eating a lot of phlegmatic foods such as tomatoes, salads, fruit juices, yoghurt and cucumber. It is a simple approach but it is very effective, and sometimes miracles happen through changing the diet.

The body itself also uses the principle of antipathy; a good example is the fever which accompanies flu. At the deepest level flu is not a viral infection, it is a disturbance of the humoral balance in the body; an excess of moisture and cold has developed. The body's natural reaction to this problem is to generate extra heat which will drive out the excess slime. Thus the fever, and the moisture, is sweated out. A natural treatment therefore would stimulate sweating and heat as much as possible, whereas an aspirin which will decrease the fever is not such a good idea. This will suppress an unpleasant symptom but will also suppress the healing mechanism. However, an excessively high temperature should be treated. Sometimes you have to deal with a dangerous or an acute symptom first before treating the deepest cause of the problem. But the beauty here is that we see the body doing what is necessary, it is the inherent wisdom of nature. Fever is not the only such phenomenon – take nose-bleeds for example. This is the body's attempt to get rid of excess blood through blood-letting in order to prevent something worse.

The counterpart of antipathy is the principle of sympathy. If you heal by sympathy you will be using remedies of the same nature as the cause, not of a contrary nature. This may be very effective and the advantage is that you need less medicine. Sympathy however cannot be applied as broadly as antipathy, there are more limitations. You will not heal a patient suffering from too much phlegm by letting him stand in the cold rain for an hour and taking up more cold and moisture. On this level the sympathy treatment does not work.

Whether sympathy can be applied depends on the kind of humor being dealt with. Adding more cold to the passive humors black choler and phlegm does not work, whereas adding more heat to the very active yellow choler does. To cool down in a hot climate you can drink something hot, Fire on too much Fire leads to decreased Fire. This is why the national cuisine of many tropical countries is extremely hot; the aim is cooling down through sympathy. If this is to work on the level of the humors there has to be a large excess of heat in the body as the cause of the disease. You can't cool so easily, but overheating does the job; there is a kind of reversal at the extreme end.

Furthermore, it depends on the level we are working at. There are two levels in treatment: the humors as the deepest cause of the illness, and the planetary energies which have become unbalanced because of the humoral excess. In the psoriasis case it is the excess phlegm which has thrown the martial energy off balance. The phlegm has to be evaporated by means of dry and hot medicine and food, but at the same time the unbalanced Mars has to be restored to its proper functioning. This can be done by antipathy or sympathy although sympathy is to be preferred, because it is more direct.

To understand more clearly how this works, we might think of a situation in normal day-to-day life. Suppose you have to deal with someone who is very angry. There are two things you can do. First you can work by antipathy. The other person is the fiery factor making a lot of noise and you will become the calming cooling factor, which tries to decrease the other person's heat. If this does not work and the other person will not listen at all, sympathy will probably be a good alternative. You confront his anger with your anger and there is a good chance that this will cool him down. Your Fire has extinguished his Fire – a nice psychological parallel to the natural physical process.

Cosmic principles

Sympathy and antipathy are cosmic principles on the basis of which we can understand how herbs have a medical effect. According to the famous seventeenth century medical astrologer Nicholas Culpeper, herbs which belong to a certain planet may work in two directions. The Blessed Thistle, *carduus benedictus*, mentioned in *Culpeper's Herbal* for example is classified under Mars in Aries and this means, he says, that it can be used against Aries and Mars diseases as well as against diseases of its opposite Venus.

This herb works against giddiness and vertigo (diseases of the head), as Aries refers to the head. It is also good against infirmities of the gall because Mars governs choler – a planet corrects that which it rules by sympathy. Mars will also heal Saturn, because Mars is exalted in Capricorn where Saturn rules. Other martial diseases against which this herb can be used are red faces, 'tetters' (skin problems), and ringworms, the biting of mad dogs and venomous beasts. However the second category consists of Venus diseases, for example the notorious French Fox or syphilis. This basic opposition Venus-Mars is even extended by sympathy/antipathy through exaltation. So a planet will be in sympathy with a planet which rules the sign it is exalted in.

This approach creates wonderful possibilities. The physical appearance of a plant shows what planetary energies it contains. It will be clear immediately that a thistle with all its thorns is a plant of Mars. On the basis of this observation only, we can conclude that the plant can be used to heal martial and venerian diseases. By classifying a plant under a planet, you know a lot about its medical properties. This is the old wisdom of the signatures, reading the planetary energies and other properties in herbs, but the same thing can be done for crystals.

It is a bit complex though, because Culpeper is often talking about planetary symbolism and much less about the humors. The planetary signature will tell you on which planetary energy the herb will have an effect, but not how; for this it has to be clear whether the herb heats or cools. To determine this, it is not enough to know the planetary symbolism. It is not always so that a plant which falls under the symbolism of Venus will be moist and cold, but it is true that a herb of Venus will balance the venerian energy stream in the body.

It is the important principle of sympathy which concerns us here on the level of the planets. If something is wrong with the kidneys, it will be a good idea to apply a herb of Venus as Culpeper states. This will support the kidney function because the kidney also falls under the symbolism of Venus. The beauty of the horary chart is that you can identify with certainty which planet has become unbalanced and so you know which kind of herbs and precious stones you will have to apply to restore the disturbed energy stream to its proper function.

An example will clarify this. Suppose we have a case of diarrhoea and the cause of the illness is given by Saturn in Cancer. Cancer is a cardinal sign and the cardinal signs move quickly. It is a Water sign involved in excretion, so we have a case of excretion happening too fast here. The excess Water of Cancer has disturbed the Saturnian function, there is little 'holding' power in the body. As a remedy we can use norit, the black coal powder that is cold, drying and very Saturnian. Norit acts on two levels.

The cold and dry coal powder introduces more holding power in the intestines. It slows the fast moving water down, especially through its drying effect. This is antipathy, but only partly so because norit is cold and the disease is also cold. Furthermore the coal powder with its Saturn signature will have an effect on the weakened Saturn energy which is part of the problem. It will strengthen the Saturn function in the body, which will be restored to its balanced state. This will also contribute to healing, as the end goal of healing is restoring the balance so that the planetary energy streams in the body will function well again. In this case we could also use Mars herbs which are often hot and dry, Mars is in sympathy with Saturn through exaltation, and its heat and dryness will further evaporate the excess phlegm.

It is a good idea to keep the sympathy/antipathy pattern in mind. We can often make good use of it, and it does contribute to a better understanding of the effects of herbs, stones and other remedies. The exact effect of herbs is not easy to predict on the basis of astrological symbolism only. They may have a primary and a secondary effect or even have different effects in different parts of the body, so some practical knowledge of the effects of herbs on certain symptoms and organs is necessary to make the picture complete. The most important point is that there are two principles in treatment: sympathy and antipathy, and that we apply sympathy mainly on the level of the planets.

Homoeopathy

A very specific use of the sympathy principle is homoeopathy. This form of healing is based on the so-called 'similia' rule: an illness can be healed by what causes it, which is the same as the ancient sympathy principle. Homoeopathy identifies the state of the patient. Through careful observation and an interview it is determined to what remedy the state of the patient corresponds. For example when he is very agitated and fiery, his state corresponds to a condition which could have been caused by the fiery poison nut, Nux Vomica.

In that case the right medicine is Nux Vomica, according to a very strict application of the sympathy principle. The hot and fiery poison nut will remove the excess fire from the body. To create this sympathetic effect the mother tincture is diluted and shaken several times, in this way the medicine receives potency. Dilution of the mother tincture of the remedy will make it purer and purer and the medicine will increasingly lose its material aspect. The further this process is continued, the stronger the medicine will be.

The principle behind the sympathy effect is simple. A purified energy will show its sympathetic effect especially strongly, and this can correct a less pure energy of the same kind. This is the same thing as teaching; someone who cannot read cannot teach this ability to a child. There has to be a higher, purer level present, which can support the lower level. Only a pure martial energy will be able to correct an unbalanced Mars which causes diseases. The homoeopathic process of dilution is such a purification so that the essence of the medicine will be able to show itself in a very pure way. The dilution of the mother tincture will remove the impure material cover, which frees its essence.

A further point of importance with regard to sympathy and antipathy is the planetary axis along which the opposites and complements work. These axes are mainly given by the oppositions of the signs. Mars opposes Venus, Jupiter opposes Mercury, and the Sun and the Moon oppose Saturn. It shows that we may use a solar medicine against a Saturnian disease (antipathy) but we may also apply Saturn itself. A good example of antipathy is the use of St John's Wort, a solar herb, against depression (Saturn), but we could also apply a Saturn stone like sapphire.

Nicholas Culpeper gives us a method to determine if antipathic or sympathetic remedies should be used. The planet that has caused the disease is compared to the planet which symbolises the diseased organ or body part. If this is the same planet you use sympathy, meaning remedies which fall under the symbolism of this planet. If the planets are different then you use antipathy. If the Sun is the cause of a skin disease, you use antipathic remedies falling under Saturn, as Saturn symbolizes the skin and the remedy will support the skin. So what you try to do is support the diseased organ by remedies of the same planetary symbolism.

As already mentioned above there is also sympathy by exaltation. A planet will support the ruler of the sign in which it is exalted by sympathy. So for example Venus will support Jupiter because Venus is exalted in Pisces, which is ruled by Jupiter. This is extended to the opposition. A planet is in antipathy to the sign and exaltation rulers of the sign in which it is in its fall, which is, however, much weaker than direct antipathy of opposing sign rulers. So Venus is in antipathy with Mercury, the exaltation ruler of Virgo in which Venus is in fall. In Virgo Mercury happens to be the sign ruler too, so this does not give another antipathy. But often planets are part of antipathy/sympathy pattern involving three other planets. The Sun and the Moon are seen as a special case because of their outspoken contrary natures.

Culpeper's idea that we should support the diseased organ with remedies of the same symbolism has its limitations. There is not always an organ which is ill and sometimes more body parts/organs are diseased, so we cannot apply this rule as a strict principle, it has to fit into the situation. Moreover, Culpeper's colleague Joseph Blagrave writes that we should use the remedies which fall under the symbolism of the planet in the chart which has the most essential dignities, a principle easy to apply. So if Jupiter in Capricorn is the illness and Venus is in Pisces you can use Venus remedies which support Jupiter through sympathy by exaltation. If you do not use this strongest planet as your remedy energy, the patient will surely die, Blagrave writes.

Sometimes we can combine all these ideas and find the planet which contains the optimal healing energy. Sometimes, though, charts are not so simple and we have to weigh the importance of several principles. The most important point will always remain that the humoral effect of the herbs you use works against the humor which is present in excess: that is the deepest cause of the disease. After that we can search for a planet which supports the diseased organ or body part and improves by sympathy or antipathy the planet which is part of the disease as the chart has shown. Sympathetic remedies will always be preferred to antipathic remedies. In this way we will be able to find a very good and effective solution in many cases.

7

Treatment

Diet

A medical astrologer will always give dietary advice and in general we can work by antipathy on this level of treatment. If there is too much coldness and moisture the best we can do is evaporate water by eating warm and dry foods. Changing diet is always the fundamental measure to be taken. Without this other remedies will have less effect. It is the basis of the whole treatment and it is always important to ask a client what he eats as many people have rather strange dietary habits. If a client who is suffering from black choler turns out to eat a lot of potatoes – a cold and dry Saturnian tuber – the solution will be simple. Stop eating potatoes! This is perhaps the crucial step towards healing. Sometimes a change in dietary habits will suffice; it is the most elegant way to fight a disease.

Traditionally, healing is not something that happens outside your life by means of chemical substance; there are times you may need to take a lot of measures and healing could take months. There are strong traditional remedies, although mild measures are always preferable at first. A traditional doctor will start with dietary advice and maybe some mild herbs if the medical situation permits. Stronger herbs are only used if the changes in diet do not work and a large excess of humor is present or if the situation is more serious. There are times like this when dietary changes will not do the job and supporting the healing process with more powerful herb remedies is a good strategy. These work on the organism at a deep level and are only applied as a second step. Foods are classified as follows:

Cold and moist foods against yellow choler excess
Beers (lighter beers), cider, cold water, egg whites, milk, soy milk, whey, soy beans, tofu, tempeh, seitan (wheat gluten), cucumbers, beans, peas,

pumpkins, melons, mangos, other fruits and fruit juices (except for grapes, blackberries, raspberries, currants, gooseberries), apples, pears (their precise effect may vary depending on the taste, sweet is warmer, sour is drier), quinces, courgettes, spinach, tomatoes, salads, young very soft cheeses (like cottage cheese), pumpkin seeds (non-salted), melon seeds, fish (except for trout), kelp and other seaweeds, veal, pork, lamb, millet, mushrooms, sunflower oil, coconut oil.

In the case of too much yellow choler: exercise and competitive sports, a short dry sauna, bathing (not too hot), little alcohol (only lighter beers), avoidance of external heat sources and strong emotions, sexual activities to cool the heat down.

Blue and green colours will decrease the amount of yellow choler, as will contact with water.

Psychologically: the Fire should be expressed through assertive behaviour, sports and competition.

Cold and dry foods against blood excess
Endives, potatoes, barley, barley water with lemon juice, vinegar, lemons and oranges (sour = cold/dry), rye, gooseberries, currants, sour apples and pears (all sour fruits) chestnuts, lentils, medlar, tamarind, chicory, sprouts, vine leaves, surrogate coffee (chicory, oak, barley), beef, green olives, cauliflower, broccoli.

In the case of too much blood: get some exercise, decrease the amount of food eaten, limit social and mental activities, take more rest, do more practical work (gardening for example), allow the body to sweat-out excess moisture in a dry sauna.

Dark colours calm down the blood excess, as does direct contact with nature and the earth.

Psychologically: rest, discipline, sobriety.

Hot and dry foods against phlegm
Peppers, onions, garlic, ginger, curry, honey, horseradish, cinnamon, nutmeg, mustard, unrefined sugar, salt, (especially sea salt), winter radish, paprika powder, dried dates, walnuts, hazelnuts, pistachio nuts, parsley, radish, carrots, fennel, leeks, parsnips, asparagus, celeriac, orange and lemon peel, aniseed, old cheeses, artichokes, pure chocolate, aubergines, black olives, salted fish, maize, red wine, basmati rice, oats, goat meat, mutton, bacon, salt meats, all hot spicy foods.

In case of too much phlegm: avoid cold, look for heat sources outside the body like a hearth fire, no bathing, no raw foods, fasting (heats you up), regular exercise to activate, don't sleep too long.

Activating colours such as bright red and gold will diminish the amount of phlegm.

Psychologically: look for emotional closeness and intimacy; cry those tears, express grief, get enthusiastic about a project.

Warm and moist foods against black choler
Egg yolks, figs, olive oil, butter, raisins, white wine (and stronger beers), basil, wheat products, spelt, turnips, pods, carrots, red beets, nut and seeds (except those already mentioned above), grapes, blackberries, raspberries, soft younger cheese, duck, chicken, wild fowl, deer, doe, sheep, rabbit, shrimps and shell fish, trout, pomegranates, ghee (clarified butter), chickpeas, coconut.

Red beet juice is strongly anti-melancholic, also spelt, wheat and white wine (which can be boiled to evaporate the alcohol).

In the case of too much black choler: not too much exercise, watch out for strong external heat or cold sources, don't work too hard, not too much discipline, enjoy social activities and parties, express yourself creatively and concretely, sexual activities increase the amount of black choler especially in men.

Optimistic colours like yellowy and orange tints work well, as does contact with wind and fresh air.

Psychologically: let go and forgive, don't be so harsh on yourself and others, life is fun.

Heat can be added to cold foods through hot spices, salt and by cooking and baking. Hot foods are colder when eaten raw or cooked lightly with mild spices.

Whole grains are better than flour which tends to acidify and produce a lot of moisture. Whole grains and legumes are energetically very balanced; salts and fats heat the body.

In general spicy, sweet and salty foods have a heating quality, while bitter and sour foods are cooling (spicy-sour is heating though).

Because heat and cold are the primary characteristics, the placement on the scale of hot/cold is most important. An organism that is cold has to be heated and one that is too hot has to be cooled down. In practice we will use mainly foods of a humoral nature, contrary to the excess humor (the principle of antipathy). Also some foods can be eaten which have the temperature as the healing element but not the same degree of moisture/dryness.

If the problem is phlegm it is best to avoid all cold and moist foods and eat as much as you can from those foods listed under hot and dry. But some foods under hot and moist can be eaten too. These foods will heat the body up, and more heat always means less moisture. As a secondary axis the moisture/dryness rate depends on the heat/cold axis to a certain extent. The right strategy depends on the precise situation; if too much moisture is the problem we mainly use drying foods.

This is the reason there are hardly any herbs which contain heat and moisture of the third degree. Third degree heat is so strong that the moisture is driven out, although there are second-degree hot and moist herbs. Sometimes a food or herb will manifest different qualities, which can be quite complex as with lemons, for example. Lemon peel is heating and drying, lemon juice is cold and dry and the fruit itself is cold and not quite as dry as the juice. The extremely sour (astringent) properties of lemon juice accounts for its cold and dry nature; the fruit itself has more moisture because of its substance.

Another example is cardamom, which will use up its explosive heat quickly and therefore only works on the upper part of the digestive system. There is also a difference between primary and secondary effects. Mint seems to cool at first, but it will in the longer run stimulate the Fire in the body. It is this secondary effect which interests us most. It is not an easy task to determine the humoral effects or planetary symbolism of herbs, as the texts are often unclear and contradict each other in the extreme. We have to use our common sense, our own observations and our practical experience.

Very generally, taste will tell us something about the nature of foods and herbs and their place on the heat/cold and dryness/moisture axis. A sharp, pungent taste is a sign of heat and dryness. Such foods or drinks can be used to drive phlegm out of the body; a ginger tea may be effective at the initial stages of a cold or flu when the body is getting into a state of phlegmatic excess. A sour taste is astringent; its movement is towards earth, so it has a cooling and drying effect, which is why it works against softening, flabbiness of tissues and loss of body fluids.

But the combination of sour and pungent tastes may also have a heating effect, as the pungent adds heat to the sour. Bitter has a cooling effect, and also dries and works against parasites and inflammations. A sweet taste is building, strengthening and heating, and salt too has a heating effect. Salt will also attract moisture because of its hot and dry nature and therefore has a softening effect in constipated conditions and on stiff muscles.

Lifestyle

There are other mild measures beside foods that we can apply to promote healing without using strong herbs or other powerful remedies. These are lifestyle measures and in some situations they can be very effective. Someone suffering from phlegm excess should not exercise too much (and I have seen such cases!). Sport and competition consumes lots of heat, and in phlegmatic conditions there is not enough heat as it is, so we should not use it all up. Fanatical exercise will maintain the diseased, unbalanced condition.

It is essential to speak to the client about his dietary habits and lifestyle. It is sometimes surprising that people do not see their strange excessive habits as a cause of their problem. Drinking twelve cups of coffee a day or living at night and sleeping during the day, has a harmful effect on health. Sometimes you will have to point out that changing such habits is necessary, otherwise treatment will not be very effective; any healing will immediately be undermined by the unhealthy life style.

There is however an important principle in our consultations: measures should be moderate. A very strict diet does not accord with the traditional spirit. The astrologer first tries to re-establish the balance in the organism through diet and lifestyle by increasing the amount of foods and activities which drive the harmful humoral excess from the body. This is a moderate long-term policy which, if it is faithfully pursued, may be very effective. It is a relatively mild adaptation of diet and lifestyle but the radical diets which have gained so much popularity in our times are quite a different thing.

An example is the raw food diet in which heating as a form of preparation is rejected. The danger is that the body will cool too much especially when people get older, or if they are by nature melancholic or phlegmatic. This is not to say that this diet will certainly lead to disease, but to maintain the heat in the bodily system, more heating herbs will have to be used. Vegetarians who eat many raw foods and moistening/cooling vegetables run this risk. In bodies which are cold by nature it may lead to an excess of cold and moisture and to the development of phlegmatic diseases.

The principle which connects lifestyle to the medical-astrological consultation is again that the client should avoid all things that increase or strengthen the humor that is the cause of the disease. If there is too much yellow choler the Fire has to be led out of the system, so intensive exercise, sports and competition will be healing. So will be contact with water; swimming is an excellent way of getting rid of excess Fire. A gentle dry sauna is also good, the heat in the sauna will drive out the excess heat in the body by sympathy, but staying in too long would heat you up.

Fasting is not good in a choleric condition as it tends to heat you up. It is excellent for phlegmatic conditions though and phlegmatics will also lose some weight then. In the case of phlegmatic excess the patient should engage in heating activities as much as he can, so no bathing, (this is very moistening). A sauna is useful but one must stay in the sauna long after the choleric has left, to really heat up and sweat out the excess moisture. Sleeping too long is not good, but moderate exercise is, as it will activate the opposite humor of Fire.

So we see different strategies on the lifestyle level: applying and activating the opposite humor by suitable activities, at the same time as expressing the excess humor to get rid of it.

In the case of excess of black choler there is not enough positive contact with life. These patients tend to eat little, which will cool them further. People who spend their days in intensive deep study may develop black choler diseases in the melancholic phase of life between forty and sixty. A regular glass of wine will work miracles, as all this serious work does not make you happy.

However, sexual activities will not be too healthy in melancholic conditions, as heat and moisture leave the body in this way, especially in men who will become drier and colder. In the case of melancholic excess we should keep as much moisture and heat in the body as we can. The Dutch writer Gerard Reve, in a deeply depressed mood, once described red wine, movies and masturbation as his main fields of interest. But as he writes, all the bottles have been emptied, there are no cinemas nearby, so life tends to become a bit monotonous. The first two activities do work against black choler, but the third will increase its excess. All the black choler in Reve's system did, by the way, lead to beautiful literature! Excess black choler can always be expressed well in artistic creations; this is the secret behind creative therapy.

If there is too much blood in the system, we need cooling and drying remedies, and from a medical perspective frequent sex is to be recommended. Discipline, concentration, hard work in isolation or in nature is also good, but wine and creamy foods should be avoided. One's agenda should not be too full; social and mental activities have to be curbed. Too much blood may be compared to an overactive steam in the body; everything that calms down this steaming is healing. Contact with the earth under one's feet is very good; gardening would be a healthy activity in the case of sanguine excess. The slow calm energy of the earth takes the heat out of the steaming blood.

Traditional psychology

Diseases also have a psychological dimension and on this level every humor has its associated measures. Too much blood requires more calming down and more discipline (in the real sense of limitation). The opposite humor of black choler requires the opposite – more looseness and streaming. Cold and dry Earth tends to freeze the psychological processes and the deepest cause is often grief or a lack of trust which results in stagnation or attempts to achieve rigid control. These are the people who still haven't forgotten what a parent or a teacher did or said thirty years ago. Forgiving is the effective medicine to defrost this chilled ice stream.

Excessively rigid life principles are also damaging to people of a melancholic nature. The more extreme Calvinist churches in The Netherlands are a good example of this gloom and spiritual hardness which actually makes people ill. But a rigid, controlling mentality can manifest in other fields of life as a result of our modern idea that we can achieve what we want if only we try hard enough.

The problem is that many people with too much black choler in their temperament feel attracted to these kinds of rigid spiritual movements or ideas about life. A sense of humour, letting go, enjoying life and putting things into perspective are the remedies. These are all things which fit the sanguine mentality, characterised as it is by airiness and casualness. We need some airiness now and then; Air will loosen up the Earth which sticks together too closely. Every gardener knows this is necessary; as inside so outside. And as we mentioned above, too much black choler demands a creative expression; the chaotic Earth is given a form and made manageable in this way.

As we saw before, if there is too much yellow choler, competition is required and the Fire is used up in exertion and tussles. Yellow choler is fast and sharp and has to get out of the system in whichever level or way that it can. In our times this is a problem because the expression of Fire is not easily tolerated and can be seen as incorrect. It is difficult for those among us who have a fiery temperament; they always hear that they are not nice or polite. This is not helpful, as in the interest of social and psychological health, Fire needs to be expressed. Controlling Fire too much will lead to Fire diseases, or to uncontrollably fiery outbursts which are unhealthy for the human system. This is not to plead for aggressive behaviour, but for more tolerance for Fire expressions which our society tends to reject. People should not feel guilty if they show their yellow choler in an acceptable, controlled way necessary for their mental and physical balance.

For its opposite humor of phlegm, streaming is required, as it is with the other cold humor black choler. But in this case it is a stream of emotions which must be expressed. Phlegm excess may be caused on the psychological level by bottled-up frustrations – a normal part of our existence. But tears that were not cried because they were seen as unacceptable can take the form of excess phlegm in the body, and may cause chronic phlegmatic diseases. Crying those unshed tears will have a healing effect allowing the excess moisture to leave the body. Also experiencing emotional intimacy and closeness is very helpful against phlegmatic disorders; the bottled-up phlegm can stream again in emotional intimacy.

Finally in sanguine disorders, calming down is required. Psychologically, blood excess points to too much enthusiasm, a constant need to connect, to communicate and do things in groups. In the case of sanguine excess, this activity should be drastically decreased. Being alone in nature is also good as groups and people are not interesting all the time, actually they can be quite boring. The addiction to communication and social activities should be replaced by a meditative, contemplative mentality which has its basis in itself. The peace resulting from this attitude will quiet the overheated organism and support the healing of sanguine illnesses.

Herbs

If mild measures do not have enough effect, herbs can be used. In the book written by Richard Saunders, *The Astrological Judgement and Practice of Physick* (1677), simple general remedies are mentioned as well complex remedies sometimes composed of many herbs and substances. These complex remedies are in most cases difficult to make, although almost all the formulas and recipes are still known. In the old days an apothecary made up these remedies, and the patients could obtain them there. Unfortunately such apothecaries no longer exist and producing these complex remedies would simply cost too much time and energy. Nevertheless there are still many simpler remedies which are effective. The way we work is as follows. First we select herbs which work against the humor in excess that has caused the disease (see list below for some examples). We may also take a look at the remedies mentioned by Saunders in his lists of planetary positions in the signs as causes of the disease; several herbs will be mentioned there. From these suggestions we make a choice on the basis of the following principles:

- the herb should work against the humoral excess that causes the disease; this is the most important thing.
- as regards its planetary nature the herb should be in sympathy, direct or through exaltation, with the disease cause or in antipathy, depending on the dignity of the planets concerned.
- try to support the diseased organ with a sympathetic herb.
- try to support Lord 1 with a sympathetic herb.
- you may add a herb of the Sun which supports general vitality.
- you may add a small quantity of a herb which is humorally in antipathy to the main herb.
- you may add a herb which works against the symptom.

In this way we can choose a single herb or a mixture on the basis of the horary chart. If Mars in Scorpio is the cause of the disease, we have to use herbs which release the phlegm and correct Mars. This is possible by applying a herb of Mars (sympathy) or a herb of Venus (antipathy), according to Nicholas Culpeper's principles. With Mars in Scorpio we would prefer sympathetic herbs though as Mars is essentially strong. In Culpeper's famous *Complete Herbal* we can find the corresponding planets under which many herbs fall. Depending on the situation we prescribe one herb or a mixture of perhaps five herbs according to all the above guidelines. These guidelines are the maximum option, and it is certainly not always necessary to make use of them all.

Herbs against humors – general

Against yellow choler: hops, violet, aloes, rhubarb, agrimony, dandelion, sorrel, water-lily, groundsel, mallows.

Against black choler: fumitory, polypody, senna, borage, lemon balm, dodder, scammony, black hellebore.

Against phlegm: elder, spurge, hyssop, thyme, briony, laurel, angelica, walnut, broom.

Against blood: shepherd's purse, horse-tail, strawberry leaves, succory, plantain, burdock.

Do not use these herbs for self-medication, always consult a competent practitioner first.

Poisonous herbs can be taken as spagyric tinctures (like hellebore) or in as homoeopathic potency (the lower potencies up to D 4). The herbs mentioned are important examples. The German astrologer Bernard Bergbauer has developed a practical computer program which gives many more herbs with their humoral effects and planetary natures. Also see the general Unani treatments below.

It is important to look at the symptoms too. We can look for herbs that work against the ailment and then select the remedies which fit the cause of the disease in the horary chart as regards humors and planetary symbolism. In this way we can find the optimal herb to work against the symptom and treat the deeper cause. Friedemann Garvelmann gives clear descriptions of the humoral effects of a selection of herbs in his book *Pflanzenheilkunde in der Humoralpathologie*.

It is striking that some herbs are mentioned as a remedy against several humors in excess. Senna for example works not only against black choler but also against phlegm and yellow choler. Fumitory is slightly hot and dry, has a Saturnian nature but can be used against black and yellow choler. Here we see the principle of sympathy and antipathy working, which can make things complex. It is difficult to fully predict the effect of herbs on the basis of theory alone; some herbs have different effects on different parts of the body. And it is also possible that the immediate, primary effect differs from the effect in the longer run, the secondary effect. Garvelmann's book gives lots of practical information about this.

There are many, many opinions about the dosage of herbs, and this also depends on the kind of herb that is given and the seriousness or acuteness of the disease. It is important to ascertain whether the disease situation is really urgent, in which case high dosages are required. The dosages used vary from roughly 3 to about 30 grams a day if dried herbs are applied as a simple herbal tea. If we use a herb for gradual recovery, 3 grams a day over a longer period will suffice. If we use a mixture of five herbs to achieve a quick result, the dosage will be 25 to 30 grams a day.

Sometimes it is necessary to treat the symptom first, and then the deeper cause. An acute inflammation or an extremely high fever will have to be cooled down initially whatever the deeper cause may be. In this way we avoid the danger of aggravating the acute symptoms with our measures against the deeper cause. For a medical astrologer in our times this will not be as important as in the old days as most of the really acute cases will be treated by a regular doctor who is better equipped for emergencies than a medical astrologer.

A herbal tea is prepared by pouring boiled water over the herbs and letting it stand covered for 10 to 15 minutes. It can then be strained and drunk, preferably three times a day. It is better to build in a pause if we use herbal teas over a longer period. So we use the tea for six days then one day we rest, and we repeat this pattern until we have achieved success.

Unani

In his book Richard Saunders often recommends that the humors should be digested before they are purged. This treatment serves as a preparation loosening the humor so that it will be easier to purge. He distinguishes between "digesters" and "purgers"; only the latter really remove the humoral excess radically from the body. Digesters are especially required if we have fixed humors indicated by a placement of the disease cause in fixed signs. Unani medicine, which we have mentioned before, gives some standard treatments for all humors. These can be applied in medical astrology, also in combination with the herbs mentioned above and the remedies mentioned in Saunders' book.

Black choler

Digesting period: 15 days

Digesters: moistening foods, melon seeds, figs, raisins, cowslip, sebestan and oxymel (a mixture of five parts honey and one part vinegar).

Another remedy for black choler which has been present in the body for a long time is a decoction of half a teaspoon each of cucumber seeds, chicory seeds, cowslip and barberry root. Put these in 2 cups of very hot water. Let it cool down and mix in 1 tablespoon of oxymel.

Purging

A simple but effective remedy is senna. Make a tea of five senna pods in one and a half cups of water, then add some fennel, mint or coriander to avoid cramps.

Compound formula: add some valerian root, anise seed and one stalk of chopped celery to the simple tea.

Another possibility is 4 senna pods in one and a half cups of water with half a teaspoon each of ginger root, balm, mint, anise seeds and rose petals.

Blood

Use a mixture of chicory seeds, lettuce seeds, coriander, rose petal, sandalwood syrup, oxymel and lemon juice.

Blood is not really "purged"; the treatment attempts to achieve a gradual decrease of the sanguine excess by cooling and drying remedies.

A most effective measure is blood-letting. Blood-letting can be accomplished by doctors working along the lines of Hildegard von Bingen's medicine, but it must be carried out at the right moment (in the week after Full Moon).

A sanguine excess may lead to an acute infection, and in this case it is strongly recommended to take antibiotics prescribed by a regular doctor.

Yellow choler

Digesting period: 3 days

Digesters: quince seeds, chicory, cucumber seeds, coriander seeds, sandalwood, lettuce seeds, cold fruits such as watermelon and vinegar (if there is coughing give chicory syrup and purslane; no quince seeds).

Digesting formula: soak 2 teaspoons of coriander in a cup of water for 1 hour; add a bit of honey, strain and drink.

Purging

A mixture of violet, plum, rose, tamarind and senna pods.

A mixture of 1 teaspoon plum pulp, some capers, half a tea-spoon each of fumitory, chicory seeds and senna leaves, add 1 teaspoon of sweet almond oil and boil in 2 cups of water for 5 minutes. Cool, strain and drink.

Phlegm

Digesting period: 9 days

Digesters: cinnamon, anise, valerian root, black raisins, cardamom, garlic, ginger.

Digesting formula #1: a quarter teaspoon each of cowslip and capers, half a teaspoon aniseed, 1 teaspoon of mint. Boil in 2 cups of water for 10 minutes, strain and drink half a cup three times a day.

Digesting formula #2: 1 tablespoon of fresh cucumber with 3 senna pods. These are soaked in a pint of hot (rose) water for an hour, then add 1 teaspoon of almond oil.

Purging

Mix a quarter of a teaspoon each of hyssop, violet and ground fennel seed, put in 3 cups of water, add 1 quarter cup of black raisins, 2 chopped dried figs and 1 teaspoon of liquorice root. Boil down to one cup, add half a teaspoon each of fresh cucumber pulp, rose petals and raw sugar, boil for 10 minutes, strain, add 1 teaspoon of sweet almond oil and take 3 teaspoons in the morning.

Mix in a cup of hot water 1 teaspoon of powdered ginger and half a teaspoon of sea salt, and drink.

After the purge a cold drink of sweet basil, honey and rose water can be given and in a case of diarrhoea, yogurt and cooked rice.

A teaspoon is about one and a half grams, a table spoon three times this quantity. A cup is half a pint, this is about a quarter of a litre.

Planetary hours

The remedies mentioned above are taken from Asian Unani medicine and they are easy to make and effective. They can be used as a part of the treatment or as a general measure against humoral excesses, in combination with dietary, life style and psychological measures. Saunders' book mentions more digesters and purgers ordered by planets in sign, but not every formula is easy to make, in fact many are not.

It is important to give the remedies at a favourable time, which can be determined astrologically. As a general rule a remedy against a certain humoral excess is taken at the moment the influence of the healing "counter" humor is strong. If we want to fight phlegm, we apply the remedy when yellow choler has most influence. To determine this, the planetary hours are used. In a Sun or Mars hour yellow choler is strong, in a Jupiter hour blood is strong, in a Venus or Moon hour phlegm is strong and in a Saturn or Mercury hour black choler is strong. It is not always that straightforward though; some planetary positions have other optimal healing hours and these are mentioned in Saunders' book.

Planetary hours can be calculated on the basis of the days of the week. The Moon is connected to Monday, Mars to Tuesday, Mercury to Wednesday, Jupiter to Thursday, Venus to Friday, Saturn to Saturday and the Sun to Sunday. The first hour of a day is ruled by the planet that rules the day; the second hour comes under the next planet given in Chaldean order: Saturn, Jupiter, Mars, Sun, Venus, Mercury, Moon, and then starting again with Saturn. Traditionally a day starts at sunrise not at midnight. So the first hour after sunrise on a Monday is ruled by the Moon, the second hour by Saturn etc. This goes on through the night until the next sunrise.

A traditional planetary hour is different from the standard clock hour of sixty minutes. A traditional day hour is one twelfth of the time between sunrise and sunset. So in winter, planetary hours during the day are much shorter than in summer. We can calculate the duration of an hour by simply dividing the time between sunrise and sunset into twelve parts and proceed in the same way to calculate night hours (between sunset and sunrise). So a Monday ends at sunrise on the Mars-day, Tuesday, which in turn starts with a martial hour.

A simple trick to check out the planetary hour quickly is given by the Placidus house system, a system based on a division of time, so every house contains two planetary hours. If the Sun is in the twelfth house, it is the first or the second planetary hour of the day. By simply dividing the house into two parts, we can see exactly which planetary hour we are in.

It is important to involve the planetary hours and the chart in the treatment but also in the preparations. Traditionally herbs were picked on an hour and a day when the planet ruling the herb would be strong. A Jupiter herb such as lemon balm can best be harvested in a Jupiter hour on a Thursday, preferably with Jupiter accidentally and essentially strong in the chart. If we process the herb alchemically into a tincture or essence, it is optimal to start this in a Jupiter hour too. The more Jupiter we have, the better it is.

The herbs that are widely available nowadays have not been picked or processed at the right planetary hours, and therefore their healing power is diminished. Mostly they are not organic either. The best thing would be to pick your own herbs at the right moment, but this is not always practicable; it means the astrologer would also be running a traditional apothecary. So in many cases we have to make use of what is offered in shops, and therefore taking the herbs at the right astrological moment will be even more important.

Blood-letting

Blood-letting, a very powerful and healthy measure, must also be carried out at the right moment so that as much as possible of the humor that causes the disease is released. The same rule applies as in digesting and purging; it should be done at a moment when the energy opposite to the humor causing the disease is strong. We can use planetary hours, but some authors also use the sign in which the Moon is placed. When we let out yellow choler the Moon should be in a Water sign.

Also it is said we cannot let blood if the Moon is in Leo. This is based on the old rule that the sign of the Moon will make its corresponding organs weaker and Leo is the sign of the heart. Blood-letting requires careful preparation. In the days before the treatment only light foods should be eaten and the patient should bathe two or three times a day. Vinegar will thin the blood further. Just before the blood-letting the patient may have a light meal and sometimes a good glass of wine is recommended.

The first days after the treatment the patient should rest to give the body time to recover. Hildegard doctors adhere to the rule that a blood-letting should only be carried out in the week after the Full Moon when the humors are not so agitated and mixed up, and a meal is only allowed if the patient is weak and might faint. In the three days after the blood-letting the patient should avoid direct sun-light or the heat of fires; for a week a special light recovery diet is followed. Blood-letting is recommended for the hot imbalances, especially for sanguine excess; for the cold diseases, a vomit is often preferred. Phlegm especially is almost never treated by letting blood.

Another method applied in many forms of traditional medicine is cupping. This is done with glass or plastic cups in which a vacuum is created. These cups are put on the skin in different places depending on the nature of the disease. In this way damaging humors are drawn out, pain can be eased, and inflammations brought to the surface away from vital organs, where they can be treated better. This traditional method, still well-known in some parts of Europe in folk medicine, is frequently used by traditional Chinese doctors and is quite simple to learn and apply. The central point is the humors and cupping can also therefore be timed astrologically. There are two varieties: one dry and one with incision and bleeding. The first method has a heating and moistening effect, the second is cooling because blood is let out.

Alchemy

Alchemy offers another possibility for effective treatment on the basis of medical charts. Through alchemical or "spagyric" processing, a herb, a mineral or even a metal can be purified to considerably increase its healing power. It is similar to homoeopathic remedies except that in the spagyric method the fixed, material part is added again to the tincture in the end. Homoeopathy works from the higher, more spiritual levels downwards, whereas in alchemical remedies the material is also present as a salt in the solution.

It is not difficult to produce an alchemical herbal tincture. The procedure is as follows. Pour 300-500 ml of grappa on 50 to 100 grams of the dried or better fresh herb and let this stand for 40 days or longer.

Strain and burn the fixed parts which are left on a gas burner until you have black ashes, then grind those ashes and continue heating till the ashes are greyish or white. Soak these white ashes in distilled water, regularly shake the solution and after a day filter and evaporate the water. Repeat this process once and add the white powder you get to the fluid tincture.

This is a simple spagyric alchemical remedy which is really powerful. To make it you only need a burner, some bottles and glass pots. Medically the tincture works like the herb, although it is more intensive and works on a broader range. The tinctures can be made at the right astrological moments and they are extremely practical because you only need a few drops a day. What is very powerful is adding the tincture to the herbal tea. If we have chosen the herb we are going to use, the tincture or essence (another spagyric product, stronger than the tincture) of the same herb can also be prescribed. If you don't make them yourself, spagyric products are for sale through the internet; one of the best companies is the German firm Spagyros.

The spagyric process is based on the distinction between the three formative principles in nature: sulphur, mercury and salt. Roughly they can be compared to the Sun, the Moon and the ascendant in the chart. Sulphur is the energy and essence which gives plant and animals their identity; the vital impulse which determines the species. It is the fiery solar principle. Mercury acts as the connective power, the lunar principle, without which connection the sulphur cannot work out on earth. Salt is the material principle which gives the sulphur-mercury connection its real form.

In herbs the essential oils or resins carry the sulphur, the alcohol carries the mercury and the material part of the planet is the salt. By pouring grappa or some other liquor on the herb the sulphur and the mercury are drawn out of the plant into the liquor. The salt that is left – the material basis – is then purified by burning or calcination. After the calcinations all the coarse parts are removed by solving and filtering in distilled water. What is left is a pure white salt, which is then added to the sulphur and the mercury.

This is, as it were, a reconstruction of the plant on a higher, purer level. The tincture is the whole plant but in a strongly purified form. Because only a pure thing can act as a remedy on an impure, unbalanced state, it is logical that this process will increase the healing power of the herb. All principles are present in the tincture, so it will affect all levels: the spiritual (Sun, sulphur), the psychological-emotional (Moon, mercury) and the physical levels (Ascendant, salt). By varying the dosage we can emphasise a more physical or a more psychological-spiritual effect. The smaller the dosage, the stronger it will work on the psychological and spiritual levels. Alchemical tinctures differ from the still purer essences; tinctures retain a humoral effect, the essences much less so. Essences will be selected mainly by planetary symbolism and the symptoms they work on. Poisonous plants should never be taken as a tincture, always as an essence.

These effects of spagyrically purified essences, which work on a higher level than the humoral level, is an important point which is undervalued in a purely humoral approach. Human beings are more than just a combination of the four humors; what makes us really human is the spiritual aspect. The model of the five elements mentioned earlier incorporates this aspect, with ether as the fifth "element" connecting us to the higher spiritual worlds. Ether has no humoral effect in the sense of heating or moistening but it is always present in the other four elements, which all, in a sense, have their origin in ether. The spagyric essences can be said to be closer to ether, more harmonised, hence their powerful effects.

8

The Spiritual Level: Hildegard von Bingen

One of the greatest doctors to emphasise the influence of the psychological and spiritual level on health is the medieval German mystic Hildegard von Bingen (1098-1179). The core of her vision is that one's spiritual attitude may contribute to the development and the healing of a disease. This vision is systematically and clearly described in the book *Die Psychotherapie der Hildegard von Bingen. Heilen mit der Kraft der Seele* by the German Hildegard doctor Wighard Strehlow. It is not modern psychotherapy based on theories of the unconscious; Hildegard wants to heal the soul through conscious spiritual choice and practice, meditation, prayer and crystals.

This came from the deep Middle Ages and Hildegard represents much of what is good about medieval Christian culture; her work is one of the milestones of this period. Although her approach is not theoretical or speculative, it can still be applied successfully. The methods described by Hildegard are effective and this can be tested in practice. Hildegard's system is based on the many visions she endured, often reluctantly and full of fear.

Hildegard's soul therapy can be connected to the medical chart through the symbolism of, among other things, the precious stones she recommends. She hardly ever explicitly refers to astrology, but nevertheless worked with the background of the humoral model and the cosmology on which classical astrology is also based. So although the link is veiled, we can make the connection between Hildegard and astrology and so make use of the spiritual power of the soul for healing.

It is important to understand that this system does not reduce diseases to a punishment for spiritual failure or as it would have been formulated in the Middle Ages, for sin. This approach, which has crept back in several modern systems of therapy and psychology in a hidden form, is too limited. We are all sinners and many of us are healthy, so that is not the point. The most important thing is that we can make use of the spiritual power of the soul, along with dietary and life style measures, herbal teas, crystals, humoral psychology and spagyric tinctures, to heal if a disease has manifested itself. The simple starting-point is that someone who chooses the good, activates more of his healing soul power.

Vertebrae and planets

The system presented by Hildegard is based on a simple diagnosis of the spinal column. We simply find which particular vertebra hurts the most and this, for example cervical-3, will be connected to a number of measures. The central premise is a pair of opposites, a "virtue-sin" polarity. Healing can be supported by actively emphasising the "virtue side". We may in our times formulate this as a conscious choice to sacrifice negative, harmful attitudes like cynicism, cowardice, anger or bitterness.

The healing strategy is built up around the 35 pairs of oppositions connected to the 35 vertebrae. Hildegard makes use of images, prayer, fasting, crystals, sauna, exercise and other activities which stimulate the development of the healing virtue. Her method can be connected to the medical consultation in two ways. The vertebral diagnosis can be carried out by a physiotherapist or an osteopath. The "virtue-sin" polarity connected to that vertebra can further be interpreted within the framework of the astrological diagnosis.

The second and more clearly astrological method is based on the planetary symbolism of the precious stones and humors. For each vertebra Hildegard recommends a crystal which supports the development of the wished-for conscious choice for the positive. Precious stones are one of the most important means to make this development possible and because each is connected to a planetary energy (see the list in Chapter 9) we can find a related planet for each vertebra. The horary chart shows the planet that has caused the disease and so we can establish which pair of opposites is in play. For example, if the chart tells us that Mercury is part of the cause of the disease, we can check all oppositional pairs for which a Mercurial stone is recommended, such as agate, emerald or aquamarine. We have to take into account all possibilities of sympathy and antipathy here, so we also check vertebra with Jupiter stones.

What we are doing here is translating the system into astrological terms and this works well enough as we can see in the descriptions of the diseases connected to the vertebra. For the diseases of the third cervical vertebra for example a heliotrope is recommended. Heliotrope will help to change an overly damaging pleasure-seeking into a more modest reticence. Heliotrope is a precious stone of a Venus/Mars nature and what could fit better than this planetary signature? We must also take into account the humoral nature of the disease if we connect vertebra and illness; pleasure-seeking has to do with phlegm, the element of desire and the lack of orientation. In this way we can connect each vertebra to a humoral excess and a planetary energy by which the medical chart can be coupled to the Hildegard system.

The vertebra system is divided into five main groups. The first four refer to anatomical zones in the body, while the last or fifth group controls the other thirty vertebrae.

In the scheme are mentioned: vertebra number – anatomical correspondence – oppositional pair – crystal and planet. The crystals in brackets are those referred to by Hildegard, according to the German therapist Michael Gienger.

Group 1-7: Cervical Vertebra

C1   eyes – earthly versus divine love – gold topaz – Sun/Jupiter
C2   hearing – exuberance/discipline – jasper/sardine (heliotrope) – Mars
C3   smelling – pleasure-seeking/modesty – jasper (heliotrope) – Mars
C4   voice/mouth – mercilessness/compassion – jasper (heliotrope) – Mars
C5   throat/bronchi – cowardice/trust in God – amethyst – Saturn/Jupiter
C6   neck/shoulders/ tonsils – anger/patience – chalcedony –Moon
C7   thyroid gland/ throat/bronchi – cynicism/zest for living – onyx (agate) – Saturn (Mercury)

Group 2: Digestive System (stomach/intestines) –
8 Thorax Vertebrae

Th 1 gullet/ windpipe/ hands – hedonism/sobriety – diamond – Sun

Th 2 heart/allergies – bitterness/largesse – amethyst – Saturn/Jupiter

Th 3 stomach/intestines/breast/lungs – malice/goodness – cornelian – Mars

Th 4 digestion/heart – lying/truth – sapphire (lapis lazuli) – Saturn

Th 5 digestion/solar plexus – aggression/peacefulness – aquamarine – Mercury/Moon

Th 6 digestion/immune system – melancholy/happiness – sardonyx – Saturn

Th 7 digestion/immune system – immoderateness/moderation – jasper (heliotrope) – Mars

Th 8 digestion/immune system – coldness/warm heartedness – emerald – Venus/Mercury

Group 3: Metabolism, Urogenital System, Immune System –
4 Thorax and 3 Lumbar Vertebrae

Th 9 digestion, urogenital system, immune system – arrogance/ meekness – rock-crystal – Moon

Th 10 digestion, urogenital system, immune system – jealousy/charity – chrysolite – Venus

Th 11 digestion, urogenital system, immune system, urinary passages – ambition/ admiration of creation – emerald – Venus/Mercury

Th 12 digestion, urogenital system, immune system, lymph system – rebelliousness/ obedience – agate (jasper) – Mercury (Mars)

L1 digestion, urogenital system, immune system, groin, back – lack of faith/faith – sapphire (lapis lazuli) – Saturn

L2 digestion, urogenital system, immune system, circulation in lower part of the body – despair/hope emerald – Venus/Mercury

L3 digestion, urogenital system, immune system, womb, bladder, knees, legs – licentiousness/simplicity – sapphire (lapis lazuli) – Saturn

Group 4: Knees, Bottom, Legs – 2 Lumbar, 5 Sacral and 1 Coccyx
Vertebrae

L4 digestion, urogenital system, immune system, hips, knees, feet – unfairness/justice – aquamarine – Mercury/Moon

L5   digestion, urogenital system, immune system – laxity/
       decisiveness – emerald – Venus/Mercury
S1   digestion, urogenital system, immune system, circulation in the
       legs – godlessness/wholeness – diamond – Sun
S2   digestion, urogenital system, immune system – instability/
       steadfastness – gold topaz – Sun/Jupiter
S3   digestion, urogenital system, immune system – care for the
       material/basic trust – sardonyx – Saturn
S4   digestion, urogenital system, immune system – stubbornness/
       change in attitude – jasper (heliotrope) – Mars
S5   digestion, urogenital system, immune system – addiction/
       freedom – diamond – Sun
Co1   digestion, urogenital system, immune system, spinal column –
       disharmony/harmony – chalcedony – Moon

Group 5: Five General Influences - Four Coccyx Vertebrae and the Cranium

Co2   controls group 1 (seven vertebrae) from C1 to C7 – lack of
       respect/respectfulness –amethyst – Saturn/Jupiter
Co3   controls group 2 (eight vertebrae) from Th 1 to Th 8 – instability/
       stability – jasper (heliotrope) – Mars
Co4   controls group 3 (seven vertebrae) from Th 3 to L3 –
       impressionability /religion – sapphire (lapis lazuli) – Saturn
Co5   controls group 4 (eight vertebrae) from L4 to Co1 – holding/
       letting go – emerald – Venus/Mercury

Cranium controls Co2-Co5, so through indirect influence
everything – meaninglessness/joy of living – chalcedony – Moon
    A very negative attitude may cause problems and a change of
attitude will contribute to recovery.

    In the Hildegard scheme most stones will be mentioned more than
once. This refers to the several effects the stone may have. In practice
there are several possibilities to choose from if you know which planet
and humor have caused the disease. A planet does not refer to only one
pair of oppositions, but because Hildegard also mentions in which part
of the body the disease connected to a vertebra manifests, it is possible
to select the right theme related to the disease on the basis of the chart.

The body is divided into four zones: the first seven vertebrae relate to the head and the senses, vertebrae eight to fifteen to stomach and intestines, the next seven to kidney, liver, sexual and other organs nearby and the next eight vertebrae to bottom and legs. The last five vertebrae are general in nature and not related to specific organs.

To illustrate how this works, we can look at the chart of the digestive problem in Part 2 where Venus in Libra turned out to be the cause of the disease. In the Hildegard system the diseased part of the digestive tract falls in the second anatomical zone. The nerves which are bundled in these vertebrae control the digestive tract. We have to look for a vertebra connected to a Mars or Venus stone, which should also fit the humoral excess and the whole clinical picture. The tenth vertebra is related to carneol which has a Mars/Venus signature and the fourteenth vertebra to heliotrope which has the same signature. Vertebra 14 is connected to the theme of 'immoderateness' versus moderation, in Latin *immoderatio* versus *discretio*. This also fits the case and the humoral excess. Blood is the expansive humor and will exceed bounds.

In the system immoderation is described as anarchy and revolution on any level, its picture is a wolf. Hildegard gives a series of measures which bring back moderation like light fasting and exercises in keeping with the right measure and the golden mean. Heliotrope can support this process, taken into the mouth it stimulates concentration and works against extreme points of view. In the book by Wighard Strehlow every vertebra is systematically related to a series of spiritual measures.

This is quite different to modern psychotherapy and the ambivalent heritage of Sigmund Freud with its one-sided emphasis on analysing the unconscious. In the traditional Hildegard psychotherapy conscious choice and cultivating the right attitude is preferred to digging into the unconscious. This is achieved on the basis of a precise knowledge of the effect of diverse measures like fasting and wearing crystals. The unconscious which was known in the tradition under another name is kept closed; real healing does not come from the unconscious astral level, but from being conscious and taking action.

This connection with Hildegard's soul therapy adds the important spiritual level to our store of healing measures, which we can recommend to our clients and whose effects should not be underestimated. In one case a harsh merciless attitude turned out to have caused a serious disease.

As soon as this point had been solved and changed to mercifulness, the disease disappeared almost immediately.

That is not to say that every disease has spiritual-psychological causes; that would be too radical. Inborn weaknesses in combination with negative progressions, the wrong diet and life style can also cause disease. What it does show is that the spiritual power of the soul can be activated to effect healing if a disease has manifested.

Analysis of the Hildegard concept:

1.   Diagnose through the medical chart the cause of the disease; a planet in combination with a humoral excess.

2.   Find the anatomical zone in which the disease has manifested and look this up in the Hildegard vertebrae scheme.

3.   Select the pairs of opposites which fit the cause of the disease (planet through sympathy/antipathy plus humoral excess).

4.   Choose from this shortlist the most probable pair of vertebrae. The nature of the humoral excess (active and exceeding bounds is Fire and Air; passive and indulgent is Earth and Water). The nature of the planet which has caused the disease and the nature of the symptoms are very important.

5.   Select the spiritual measures which relate to the vertebrae and the connected "virtue-vice" pair as part of the astromedical consultation. The book by Wighard Strenlow which was mentioned in the first paragraph of this chapter gives a whole range of further possible measures for each "sin-virtue" pair.

9

Precious Stones

Lucifer's crown

As we have seen in the preceding chapter it is Saint Hildegard von Bingen who leads us in the right direction if we think about the mysterious power of crystals. The mystic and prophetess from the 12th century was not an astrologer, but there is often much more we can learn about our celestial art from mystics, theologians and mythology than from astrologers themselves. This is also true of the way Hildegard writes about the essential nature of precious stones.

She says that precious stones were originally set by the Almighty in the crown of his most powerful servant, the Angel of Dawn, Lucifer. But as we know, this elevated position was too much for the Light-bearer and he rebelled against God's authority because he did not want to serve. The first sin was born and although Lucifer was able to seduce one third of the angelic armies to his side, he eventually lost. No one can stand against the Almighty and win; a rebel has no chance. Lucifer was punished for his rebellion and thrown down into hell with his allies and became Satan. His angelic allies in the battle against the Light have been crippled into a dark army of unhappy demons, who will plague humankind until the end of time. The former Angel of Dawn had to forfeit his crown before being thrown into the darkness of Hell and the precious stones set in the crown were now destined for man by God.

This mythical story told by Hildegard shows that a very pure energy is captured in precious stones, which has its origins in the pure world which existed before the fall of the Angel of Dawn. It shows that precious stones are essentially pure energies which can be used to correct a less pure or disfunctioning energy. This is one of the ways Hildegard uses them, as instruments which lead mankind to its better and lighter side.

Emerald for example helps in changing despair into hope and sardonyx in changing depression into merriness. To put it briefly: crystals bring out the best in you. We can use them in connection with the medical horary chart, among other things through their associated planetary symbolism.

Precious stones can be compared to planets with essential dignity, brought into tangible form. A ruby is more or less the Sun in Leo so can be used to strengthen the solar energy; its pure energy will raise a weak solar energy on to a higher level. Every stone is 'signed' in this way by planetary forces; the planets inscribe the stones with their energy. This is the stone's signature which manifests in its effects, colour, the site where it is found and other characteristics. The signature will make clear to which planet the stone belongs, although this requires experience, caution and care; it is not always immediately clear.

There are stones which are assigned to two planets and so have a mixed signature, which can be confusing. It is one reason that sources tend to contradict each about the signatures of precious stones. Also differently coloured varieties of the same stone may fall under different planets. In Vedic astrology the blue sapphire is a stone of Saturn and the yellow sapphire is a Jupiter stone. This shows that both planetary energies work in the stone but its colour points out which energy is the strongest.

As mentioned above the planetary symbolism allows us to use precious stones on a much broader scale on the basis of the medical horary. We can go much further than just the stones Hildegard describes in her vertebrae system with the spiritual diagnosis, for every stone for which we can establish a planetary link can be used for healing. The medical horary shows which planetary energy stream is out of balance according to which humoral excess, and so we can correct this imbalance by means of an appropriate stone.

Signatures

To let the whole system work in an acceptable way we must establish which planets work in which precious stones. The planets are the dynamic powers which give form to our reality and their 'impression' can always be seen in concrete objects. In herbs we can also recognize the signatures in this way; St John's wort is a solar plant and can therefore heal depression. However in herbs, signatures tend to be more strongly mixed, and it requires a lot of experience to recognise them in their proportions.

Fortunately, precious stones are clearer. Sometimes we see mixed signatures but not such complexity as with herbs; in many cases there is clearly one planet which determines the stone's effects. This is logical because stones have a totally different nature; they were placed in Lucifer's crown, whereas herbs are more a part of the whole seasonal cycle on earth, the world of growth and decay. Stones distinguish themselves by their pure, stable and balanced character, as Hildegard emphasises.

So establishing the planetary nature for a stone is easier than for a herb and we can use different methods to find the right planet. Firstly we have the traditional texts in which planets are coupled to precious stones. They must be taken seriously, but also critically read. The dogmatic point of view that everything that was written down in the past by someone is absolutely, literally true will not lead to an effective and practical traditional astrology.

Secondly, it is important to look at the effects of stones, to base your knowledge on your own experience and on the texts of modern stone therapists. A good modern expert is Michael Gienger who writes clearly about the effects of stones; his ideas are based on experience and practice. The next thing is to judge the stone, to determine if its colour, characteristics and whole appearance fit with a particular planet. In this way we can usually discover to which planet the stone is assigned

To show how this works, let us look for example at a blue chalcedony. In traditional astrological texts it is not mentioned very often, but in the Hildegard system it is very important. The effects of the stone are, according to several authorities, said to strengthen the power of speech ("orator stone"), and to bring calmness. It works on the mucous membranes and the lymph and other body fluids; it improves the secretion of hormonal glands, it lowers the blood pressure and stimulates milk production in nursing mothers. To put it briefly, we have a stone here which lowers the energy level, calms us down and is strongly connected with fluids.

Furthermore chalcedony is relatively soft and its main tints are a lovely pink, blue and white. Now we critically look at all the seven planets until the right one is found by a process of elimination. It is not the Sun or Mars, because of the calming and fluid nature of the chalcedony. For Jupiter it is too calm and too soft in colour. For Saturn it is too lovely and too related to fluids. With Venus we get nearer, but Venus' colour is mostly green and chalcedony lacks the typical effects of Venus.

This leaves us with the Moon and Mercury. Chalcedony is known as the orators' stone; even stammerers will speak with more ease with the help of this stone or its essence. This seems to point into the direction of Mercury, but chalcedony does not really have an overall Mercurial signature, which would show itself as a large variety of forms or a very outspoken layered structure, (as with agate for example). Neither is Mercury much connected to streams of fluids. So this leaves us with the Moon, and this planet seems to fit perfectly with the calming, soft and fluid nature of chalcedony.

But why would a Moon stone like chalcedony be known as the orators' stone? This is because Mercury is fed by the Moon. Traditionally the Moon is the mind and the inspiration, Mercury only the channel through which it is expressed. If you want to improve your oratory capacity you could use a Mercury stone like emerald or aquamarine, but with chalcedony we are on a deeper level. When the Moon functions well, there is inspiration, the stream of words flows abundantly – Mercury is fed by the Moon which connects it to the Sun, the spiritual source of truth.

The lists below were developed on the basis of the method. This scheme has been tested, although in some case there may remain doubts, especially when two planets work in one stone. If there is a second planet, this is mentioned in brackets.

Planetary signature of precious stones

Saturn: calcite, obsidian, galenite, antimonite (Mars), chiastolite, lepidolite, charoite, amethyst (Jupiter), lapis lazuli (Jupiter), sapphire, sardonyx (sarder-onyx combination: Mars), charoite, smoky quartz, tiger's eye, hawks' eye, sugilite, pietersite (crocidolite), cerrusite, iolite, petrified wood, black tourmaline, halite/stone salt (Mars), apatite (Sun), jet, fluorite, sphalerite, aragonite.
Metal: lead
Colours: all dark tints.

Jupiter: turquoise (Moon/Venus), topaz, larimar, moldavite, dumortierite, cassiterite, zircon.
Metal: tin
Colours: sky blue, purple, bluish green tints.

Mars: hematite, jasper, heliotrope, vivianite, magnetite, tiger iron, mookaite, carneol (Venus), sard (Venus), garnet, rhodonite, moqui marbles (eagle stone).
Metal: iron
Colours: red, iron colour.

Venus: serpentine (Moon, Mars), chrysocolla, chrysoprase, dioptase, malachite, azurite, nephrite, jade, epidote (Mars), peridote (Mars), rose quartz, aventurine, actinolite, thulite, rhodochrosite (Mars), opal (Mercury), prase, coral, amazonite, emerald (Mercury), alexandrite.
Metals: copper, nickel, manganese.
Colour: green

Mercury: emerald (Venus), beryl, aquamarine (Moon), opal (Venus), agate, tourmaline (special case, see below), cinnabar, kyanite, flint, feldspar.
Metal: quicksilver
Colour: varying, many-coloured.

Sun: amber, citrine, ametrine, (citrine/amethyst combination, also Saturn), chrysoberyl, pyrite, pop rocks, chalk pyrite, ruby, orthoclase, sun stone, spinel, topaz imperial, rutile quartz, variscite, diamond, barite.
Metal: gold
Colours: yellow, gold, orange.

Moon: pearls, moonstone, rock crystal (Sun), chalcedony, hiddenite, kunzite, labradorite, gypsum (Mars), moss agate, morganite (Venus), calcite, dolomite, apophylite, blue quartz, prehnite, anhydrite, magnesite, celestine, biotite.
Metal: silver
Colours: silvery, white, light blue, pink.

It is important to realise that one of the reasons precious stones can be distinguished is that their planetary signatures are all different. They would be much the same if they each contained exactly the same proportions of planetary forces. As they are clearly different their difference in planetary nature and other characteristics can be formulated in astrological terms. So all stones under Mars differ in nature because of the different proportions of martial and other planetary forces they contain, although some other factors like the principle of formation are also important.

Hematite with its iron-like appearance and its strongly heating effect (this stone may worsen inflammations) is dominated by Mars. Carneol, however, (red-orange colour, activating, haemostatic) also contains Venus energy; William Lilly in *Christian Astrology* mentions the stone under Venus. This is not totally correct because Mars remains the stronger energy of the two. With Mercury we see variety reaching its maximum, which might be expected from a planet whose nature consists of connections, changes and flexibility.

There are for example many, many varieties of agate which also have – through their Mercurial nature – a whole range of medical effects. The reason for this is that a specific agate variety is also influenced by another planet. Because Mercury flows along so easily, this secondary planet is able to manifest in connection with other energies, but it does not mean that the stone will lose its Mercurial nature.

To say more about the agate's effect you can look at the further signature, its appearance. Eye agate which looks like an eye will work on the eyes; fire agate is good against flu because it stimulates healing fevers (the fever's fire evaporates the excess phlegm which is the cause of the disease) and water agate is good for the womb. The agate varieties are recognised by the other energies which give them their characteristics and specific effects.

Tourmaline is a difficult case. There are many varieties of tourmaline and in Vedic astrology they are ascribed to five different planets on the basis of their colours. In this stone the Mercurial quicksilver character reaches its summit; the stones are dominated by other planets, for example black tourmaline by Saturn. The traditional Arabic ascription of tourmaline to the Sun is also confusing and might apply to the rainbow tourmaline which contains all colours like the Sun.

It is striking that the stone that works strongly against MS and palsies is watermelon tourmaline. MS is a cold and dry disease of the nervous system (Mercury): this tourmaline variety clearly contains strong Mercurial powers which can strengthen the nervous system.

In practice we choose a healing stone on the basis of various criteria. Firstly, the stone should have a colour in antipathy to the excess humor which causes the disease. In a case of too much phlegm: red activating stones; in a case of too much Air: dark inhibiting stones; too much Fire: green or blue stones and too much black choler: yellow light coloured stones. Sometimes we can also use sympathy; the dark blue lapis lazuli works against black choler, so don't take this principle too rigidly. Secondly and more importantly the planetary energy in the stone should work antipathically or sympathetically on the planet which is a part of the disease cause as given by the horary chart. This is the main criterion.

Thirdly the cross should fit the principle of formation of the stone. Primary stones, formed immediately out of the lava, correspond to the cardinal cross; secondary stones which are formed in erosion processes correspond to the fixed cross, and tertiary, metamorphous stones to the mutable cross. A good book on precious stones will give you this information. The fourth point is the symptomatic effect, and if all these four factors fit together we have found the optimal stone, although this choice should not be based on the symptoms alone.

We need to be flexible so we can combine traditional and modern texts, appearances, colours, experience and observations into an acceptable planetary signature. This does not work infallibly and there will probably be some changes to the scheme above but it is a good basis for effective consultations.

Planetary axis

The signatures often work according to the pattern of antipathies and sympathies: Venus-Mars, Mercury-Jupiter, Sun-Saturn and Moon-Saturn. These oppositions are very important in the medical applications. Take for example heliotrope, a Mars stone also ruled by Venus. It can be used to diminish martial heat but also to burn away a lack of energy (phlegm) through its martial power. This can be checked out in practice because the stone works against slime in the sinus cavities (sinusitis) but will also calm the heart by taking away excess yellow choler which may lead to heart palpitations. If we use this stone for this purpose, it will become hot.

A precious stone can be used (according to the principle mentioned by Culpeper) against diseases in which its 'own' planet is involved and against diseases of the planet in antipathy. Even sympathy by exaltation will work; heliotrope (Mars) stimulates the immune system (Saturn), because Mars is exalted in Saturn's sign Capricorn. The best choice depends on the exact situation in the chart. If we have a very hot Mars in Sagittarius as the cause of the disease, we should always give moist and cold foods plus herbs to put out the Fire. If the Fire is balanced Mars will function well again. The reason it is not functioning as it should is the excess of yellow choler, as its Sagittarius background shows.

But we can support the healing process by correcting the martial energy. This could be achieved by means of sympathy, by a stone of Mars. But if we use a very martial stone like hematite this may not work well so it would be better to mix in some cooling Venus energy, for example a heliotrope. The stone could also be further selected by colour; if its dominant tint is green it will be more cooling. We can choose the optimal stone on the basis of the medical horary by taking into account the sympathy/antipathy patterns, colours and mixed signatures.

The basic principle remains healing through sympathy/antipathy with the deeper cause of the disease; this has a correcting and healing effect on the unbalanced planet. It is the idea of purity again; precious stones are pure so they can restore the diseased planet to its balanced state. In the end all diseases have their origin in a planetary energy which has become unbalanced as a result of some excess humor. In healing, sympathy is preferred (correcting Mars with a Mars stone), as the direct approach it is more powerful than antipathy, but we have to consider several factors. If the disease is caused by an essentially weak planet we would do better to work though a more powerful antipathic energy.

The choice of the right stone can be based on a somewhat broader interpretation of sympathy/antipathy. A cooling stone of the Moon will also work against the heat of Mars. There is also a clear antipathy relationship between cold and dry Saturn and the optimistic warm and moist energy of the Great Benefic Jupiter. So the humoral nature of the planets has a role to play. Sympathy/antipathy also works by exaltation;

a planet will work though sympathy on another planet in the sign of which it is exalted (for example Venus on Jupiter). Most important of all is to be flexible and apply the systems and schemes creatively with common sense. Precious stones are different from herbs, the focus is very strongly on the planetary energy, while herbs are characterised much more by their humoral effect.

Applications

There are many ways to bring the energy of precious stones into the body/mind system. The stones work mainly through direct skin contact; if you wear a ring or a bracelet without this contact they will not have so great an effect. A precious stone can also be laid on the body every day for a certain amount of time, which is practical especially if we want to create a local effect in some body part. If we want a more psychological or spiritual effect we can use precious stones without direct contact for meditations. It is sufficient to look intensively at the stone in a relaxed atmosphere for about fifteen minutes; looking at an object is always an exchange of energy.

Essences of precious stones are also useful. These are simple to make – the precious stones are washed and put in a glass with liquid, then covered. If water (low-mineral content, glass bottles!) is used, overnight immersion is enough and the water can be drunk the next morning, (don't do this with antimonite, azurite, malachite, Eilat stone, galenite, fluorite). The stone's energy will be transferred to the water. However we can not keep this water too long as it will soon lose its energy. If we produce the essence with alcohol, we can keep it for a longer time and this is very practical; it is possible to build up a whole apothecary of essences which are ready for use.

A stone can be put in brandy or grappa for a few months and these essences can be kept in small bottles. By also immersing a rock-crystal in the fluid, the energy of the stone essence can be further strengthened. Even more practical is the Vedic method. The stone is first washed in milk, then in clean source water, and then put into 90% pure alcohol for about 12 hours. The glass in which it is kept should catch the daylight. After 12 hours the essence (or tincture) is ready to be used. These tinctures are strong; only a few drops are required to have some effect. There are also alchemical stone tinctures, which have an even stronger effect. The fewer drops that are taken, the less physical the effects will be.

Case

It is time now to return to the charts of medical questions discussed in Part 2 to show how a medical consultation is drawn up. The question about the psoriasis showed that excess phlegm was the cause of the problem. The first measure always concerns diet; the client should eat as much of the hot and dry foods mentioned in the list in Chapter 7 and avoid moist and cold foods. She may also eat some warm and moist foods, but not too many of these because moisture is part of the problem.

For the client this was a great change. A Chinese doctor had recommended moist and cold foods some years before but this had strengthened the disease. Maybe the advice was right at the moment it was given, but the cold diet was not effective any more; the body had become too cold and moist. The effect of the switch to hot and dry foods was an almost immediate success, the spread of the psoriasis was halted and the lack of energy disappeared. Lack of energy is typical for phlegm excess. Moreover this client exercised fanatically. This also had to be curtailed as sports uses up Fire which we need to evaporate the phlegmatic excess. The chart also shows this fanatical exercise clearly in the symbolism of Mars (exercise) in a Water sign (exhaustion).

Because the problem was worsening acutely and because the prognosis (no measures taken) was not positive, a herbal tea was also recommended. She could have followed the Unani method, but Saunders also mentions some heating and drying herbs such as thyme, parsley (root), nettle and wormwood. In this case we prefer sympathetic Mars herbs like parsley and nettles because Mars is strong in the chart and nettles work healing on the skin. Specifically for the skin, fumitory can be prescribed. This Saturnian herb is good for the skin and subdues the symptom of the fiery martial energy. With this herb we strengthen the diseased organ and follow Culpeper's idea of supporting this organ by using a sympathetic herb.

We can further strengthen the effect of the treatment by spagyric tinctures of the herbs mentioned, for example a tincture of nettles as a heating herb of Mars. Another beneficial remedy for the skin, very good in cases of skin disease, is propolis. This is a kind of resin produced by bees from poplar buds which they use to close and protect their hives from infection; in effect a kind of second skin. As a spagyric essence it is absolutely safe and it may work miracles.

We can also prescribe precious stones. The problem in this case is Mars so we look for a stone on the Venus/Mars-axis. We could select a blood jasper or heliotrope which has a mixed Mars/Venus energy and combines the correction of the martial energy stream with Venus' cooling effect; it is not a very hot stone. Here we work on two levels at the same time, the heliotrope's martial energy corrects the unbalanced Mars, but the Venus energy subdues the fierce martial outbursts of fanatical exercise and a sometimes overly assertive reaction.

The Hildegard diagnosis was also carried out and most painful was the sixth cervical vertebra. This vertebra's theme is *ira-patienta*: anger versus patience. Dead on target! Hildegard's image is a rattling skeleton running in a treadmill which clearly mirrors my client's fanatical exercising. The unbridled (phlegm) "ira" (Mars) gives rise to the disease, the anger turning back on the body itself. Hildegard mentions skin diseases with peeling as a symptom of this anger. Measures are: a ten-day fasting cure during which the patient is clad in simple clothing; brush massages, showers with chestnut extracts and the conscious development of more patience.

As the stone which supports this process, a blue chalcedony is mentioned. This has a strong calming effect and is related to fluids in the body. The chalcedony will help to diminish the anger while correcting the body's water balance. So the stone works on the planetary energy as well as on the humoral balance and it is very suitable in this case. The chalcedony may be combined with the heliotrope, perhaps with the heliotrope as a necklace and the chalcedony as an alchemical tincture or essence.

In the same way we can draw up a whole series of healing measures if other humors and planets are the cause of the problem; remedies are employed on diverse levels. We fight the disease with diet, herbs, precious stones, alchemical tinctures, alteration of the life style, psychological insights and spiritual exercise. This is all systematically based on the analysis of the horary chart of the medical question, and the wide selection of treatments considerably increases the chances of healing.

PART 4

OPERATIONS

ELECTIONS

AND PREVENTION

10

Questions on Operations and Treatments

Mars, the surgical knife

In the astromedical practice questions are also asked about the treatments and operations proposed by doctors. These kinds of questions can be answered very precisely and in this way medical astrology can help patients avoid unnecessary surgery. A clear case was discussed in Chapter 5; an operation which was seen as urgent was postponed by a client after an astrological consultation. The astrological timing was correct, and three months later my client had recovered without the operation.

Astrology provides us with insights into the effects of a treatment or an operation. Very important in these questions are the receptions between the relevant planets in the chart, which show the effects of the operation on body and illness. If a question is asked about a treatment, this is always indicated by the ruler of the tenth house. If the question only concerns an operation we look at Mars. This applies to laser treatments as well as knives, as a laser beam will also cut, so we have a Mars signature there.

In analysing these charts we look at the power and effect of Lord 10 or Mars. What we like to see is a lot of essential dignity, which would show a powerful treatment. The less dignity, the less power we have. Mars in detriment in the twelfth house will probably not do much good; the operation is simply too weak, but if the placement of the planet suits the situation, negative indications may fall away. If the question above had been about the feet, then the twelfth house as the house of the feet would have shown an operation in the right place.

More important than dignity is the relationship through reception and disposition with the ruler of the first house; the crucial question is 'what effect will the treatment or the operation have on the physical condition?' This is shown by the ruler of the first house. If the significator of the operation is in negative reception with Lord 1 it will damage the body and the operation should not be carried out. Of course, we always have to consider the whole situation about which the question is asked. Sometimes we simply have little choice and we have to accept that the body will be harmed.

Disposition is also very important. Disposition shows the power that one planet has over another. If Lord 1 is in the sign or exaltation of Lord 10, the treatment has power over the body, a very positive sign. In the analysis of the network of receptions and dispositions we may also involve the cause of the disease. Of course it is favourable if the treatment has power over the disease or is in strong mutual reception with it. Its influence on the disease is favourable in that case.

Lord 1 and Lord 10 or Mars remain the main factors we have to analyse, otherwise it will become too complex. A good example would be Lord 10 which disposes the cause of the disease but at the same time receives Lord 1 into fall. The treatment has power over the disease which is good, but the body will also be harmed by the treatment. This fact is most important, although we have to decide on the basis of the whole situation if we should carry out the treatment despite its negative effects on the body.

A special case was discussed in chapter four, Part 2 of this book: the question about the acute osteoporosis caused by too much activity of the parathyroid gland, which was caused in turn by too much yellow choler. The question was also if the operation proposed by the doctors would be a good idea. In the chart Mars would be the significator of the operation. However, Mars is already in use as Lord 1 and we have to find another operation significator, as we have to distinguish between body and operation. This could be Lord 6 (the sixth house being the place where we employ the knife to fight the disease), but this is also Mars. Another possibility is the Part of Surgery/Treatment. In a day chart this part is calculated with the formula Asc + Saturn − Mars; in a night chart the formula is reversed (Asc + Mars − Saturn). The distance of arc between Mars and Saturn is projected from the ascendant and the Part falls in the eleventh degree of Libra. The Part's dispositor will serve as the operation significator, so Venus is the operation. We have to analyse the effect of Venus on Lord 1 of the body.

Venus is in Cancer, in which Mars is in fall and has triplicity dignity. So the operation (cutting out the parathyroid gland) will have a strongly negative effect on the body (negative reception through fall) but also a weaker positive effect (positive reception through triplicity). If possible the operation should not be carried out, because it will harm the body more than it will help. It would be better to try to heal with natural remedies first. It is striking that the operation's significator (in this case Venus) will soon enter Leo, so it will follow Mercury, the cause of the disease. This is not very positive at all. It will do the same thing as Mercury, which has caused the problem by its entry into fiery Leo. So the operation, if it is carried out, will have the same damaging effect as Mercury. This is another indication that the operation is not a good solution; as long as there are other possibilities for treatment these are definitely to be preferred above an operation which will have a strongly negative effect.

Treatment

A good example of an analysis of a treatment is the following chart. The problem is a chronic sinusitis which was treated with antibiotics and cortisone. This is only treating the symptom, and as the inflammation kept coming back the doctors prescribed heavier and heavier dosages. The question was asked by a mother about her child and so the child's health condition is given by the fifth house (children fall under the fifth house). This is the Moon in Pisces. We call this "turning the chart". If someone asks a question about another person we look at the house which represents this person and we work from that house.

So we have a planet in a sign fitting its humoral nature, the Moon is cold and moist and Pisces is cold and moist. It means the Moon's dispositor is not necessarily the cause, but we can take Jupiter as the cause of the disease here because Jupiter is in negative reception with the Moon, which has its fall in Scorpio. The placement in Scorpio, a fixed sign, points to a considerable excess of fixed phlegm which fits the whole picture. The Moon's last aspect with the Sun indicates the inflammatory nature of the disease. This is however not the point here; the question is

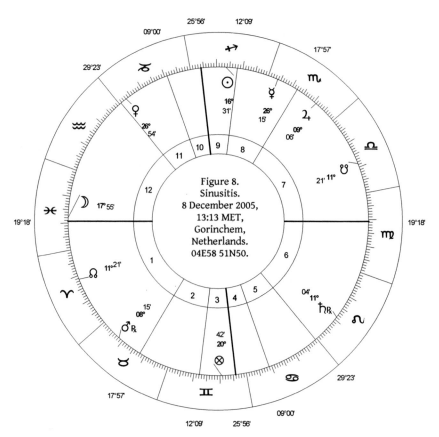

Figure 8.
Sinusitis.
8 December 2005,
13:13 MET,
Gorinchem,
Netherlands.
04E58 51N50.

whether the treatment is good. Lord 10 is Venus in Capricorn, ruler of the tenth house counted from the fifth house of the child, and shows the treatment the child is receiving. What is the effect of this Venus on Lord 5? Lord 10 receives the Moon into detriment (the Moon is in detriment in Capricorn) and so has a damaging effect on the body. However, Venus is the exaltation ruler in Pisces and so the treatment has power over the body.

Although the treatment removes the symptoms effectively, it does not heal the disease. The treatment even cools the body more and more and in this way it maintains the illness. Venus in Capricorn, a cold planet in a cold sign, is not the right remedy for a cold disease. Moreover the ruler of the turned tenth house takes the Moon into detriment, so damages the body and it is in a negative harming reception through fall with Jupiter in Scorpio, the cause of the disease. The situation improved as a result of the astromedical consultation, which is not surprising with a view to the effects of Lord 10 on the body. Heating and drying herbs and foods were successfully used to evaporate the excess slime.

11

Medical Elections

Horary elections

Another possibility which medical astrology offers is making elections for an operation, a cure or a treatment. We can choose the most favourable time for the start of an operation or a course of treatment. The client simply asks for the best time to undergo an operation. This is relatively simple as the significator of the operation in the chart is moved forward to its optimal position. The distance to this position in degrees can be converted into the right time units, which will mostly be weeks or months.

The horary chart is so practical because it indicates the time roughly and not necessarily exactly. Of course we could also calculate an exact full election chart, but this is problematic for treatments for which doctors are required because electional charts are calculated to the minute and a few minutes later the most favourable time may be over. To be able to use full elections the client has to have complete control of the situation. Only then can he exactly determine when it starts. Almost the only time this can work is with treatments in which pills are taken.

If a full election is calculated we must refer to the natal chart or the election will be unreliable and even potentially dangerous. Suppose we elect a chart and in this chart we have Lord 1 and 10 (body and treatment) in a strong positive mutual reception or dispositional relation. This seems to be fine, but we also have to look at the planet which is Lord 1 in the natal chart. In most cases this will not be the same planet, and the planet positions in the election chart might even be damaging to natal Lord 1.

It means that the client's body would be harmed by starting the treatment at that moment; calculating an election chart without involving the natal chart is not effective and this also applies to non-medical elections. Elections based on the position of the Moon are also imprecise and do not have much practical value. The idea behind the Moon election is that the organ corresponding to the sign in which the Moon currently is placed is extra vulnerable – so stomach operations should not be carried out when the Moon is in Cancer.

There is not much value in this idea and it is better to use horary charts which are not too much work and are much more precise. Do not make the mistake of checking the time you have calculated by means of the horary election chart in the ephemeris. If you do that you have slipped into calculating a full election again! A horary is a complete universe in itself, you don't need to refer to another chart to find the answer (and this is also true outside of medical astrology).

A clear example of an election question is the following case. The client is scheduled to have an operation to remove a benign tumour and she asks whether the operation will have harmful effects and if the scheduled time is favourable. Would it be a good idea to postpone it? This is a double question, about the effects of the operation and about the best moment. In the chart the operation is Mars, which is also clearly indicated by the Moon on the sixth house cusp (the house of the surgical knife) which is ruled by Mars.

Firstly, the effect of the operation. Mars is placed in Libra, the sign ruled by Venus/Lord 1 (the body) and although it has no power over Venus, it is in positive reception with the body. The operation will not harm Venus because it is in the sign of Venus. The ascendant is on Spica, a powerful and favourable fixed star which gives protection, and this is an indication that all will end well. Technically, Mars is in the first house (being within a five degree orb from the house cusp) and not in the vague, harmful twelfth house. The fact that Mars is in detriment in Libra does not count as negative because Libra anatomically corresponds to the womb, the organ which will be operated on. The knife is in the right place.

All in all very positive. The conclusion is that the operation will have little negative effect. Now we look at the timing. The operation is planned for 2nd November; the question is if there is a more favourable

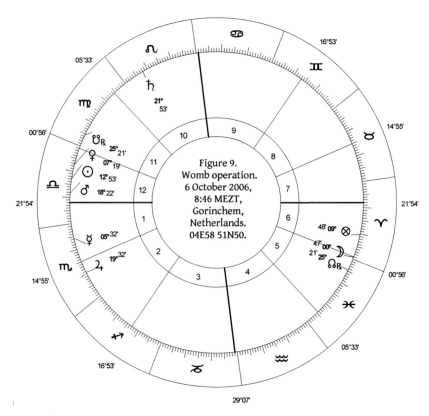

Figure 9.
Womb operation.
6 October 2006,
8:46 MEZT,
Gorinchem,
Netherlands.
04E58 51N50.

time for the operation to take place. If we move Mars forward somewhat more than three degrees (1 degree = 1 week), this corresponds to the scheduled time, it will be exactly on the ascendant and exactly on Spica. Splendid! The operation in conjunction with the body is fine. If we move Mars further, we see no improvements. The Sun will come nearer and nearer and Mars will be increasingly combust which will weaken it. A combust significator of the operation is not a good idea; combustion is blinding so the surgeon would not have all the necessary information at his disposal. Mars will enter Scorpio after some time, but this will not make it better, it will receive Venus, the body, into detriment there and this is not good. The best time is the one scheduled; this would have been the time we would have recommended on the basis of the election question.

The operation was carried out successfully at the time planned. The only thing that worried me me to some extent was the exact sextile of this nasty Saturn in detriment in Leo in exact sextile with the ASC-degree, a minor point but it did not look too good. The operation left a very, very large scar!

Two cataract operations

This question was asked by a client who was to have a cataract operation and he wanted to know the optimal time. The most important principle of an election horary is to make the relevant significators as strong as possible. Because it concerns surgery on the eye, we have to look at Mars as the knife and the Sun or the Moon as the planets that symbolize the eyes. As the client is male and the operation is to be carried out on the left eye, the Moon is of great importance, in males the Sun is the right eye and the Moon the left eye.

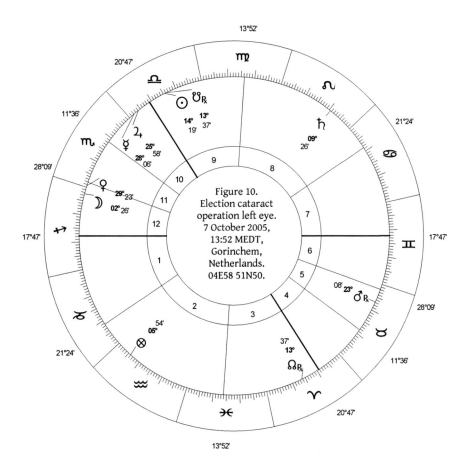

Figure 10.
Election cataract operation left eye.
7 October 2005,
13:52 MEDT,
Gorinchem,
Netherlands.
04E58 51N50.

We can see this in the chart of the question "When is the optimal time to have this operation?" The Moon as the significator of the veiled eye is on the cusp of the malefic twelfth house of disappearances, and the Moon is on the fixed star Yed Prior of a Saturn/Venus nature. Fixed stars describe a situation further and here the Saturn symbolism stands for the corneal hardening. The constellation Yed Prior is part of Ophiuchus which refers to medicine.

The other eye, the Sun, is also weak in conjunction with the South Node (also Saturn-like) and in detriment in Libra. Later the client was also due an operation on the right eye, but the left eye which was worse was to be treated first. In an election we are looking for the most favourable time so we move the relevant significators forward to their optimal positions. It is clear that the Moon should be out of the malefic twelfth house if the operation takes place. A good place is on the ascendant, the significator of the eye strong in conjunction with the place that symbolizes the body would be good.

If we move it further we bump into Pluto, which can be seen as a fixed star of a special kind with a very malefic nature. The region that comes after Pluto at the end of Sagittarius is not safe either because here we find the fixed stars Aculeus and Acumen. These stars are nebulous star clusters; not a good sign for clear sight. The next sign Capricorn is unfavourable as the Moon will be in detriment there in opposition with its own sign Cancer. The only place favourable for the eye is on the ascendant, about fifteen degrees measured from its position in the chart.

This is important, but we should look at other relevant factors too, such as Mars as the natural significator of the surgical knife. Mars does not look good at all in its detriment in Taurus and retrograde. It seems to suggest that the operation should be postponed for a longer period of time, but this would hardly be possible with a view to the worsening medical situation. Moreover, Mars' detriment is not too bad for it is in the exaltation of the Moon, so Mars (the knife) will not harm the eye (Moon). This means we can disregard its detriment; the knife is in the place we would like to find for an eye operation although it could of course be more favourably placed. Its retrogradation will remain problematic, but we cannot do anything about it within the time period given by the Moon's favourable positions. Sometimes this happens, and we have to work with the timing that is available.

Mars in the exaltation sign of the Moon does give us a warning. Mars' surgical knife exalts the eye, meaning that the knife 'sees' the situation of the eye a little too rosily. This is always the meaning of exaltation; we often see this reception in horary questions about love. So I told the client to ask his doctor to be extra careful and to check that nothing is over-looked. If a doctor would take such a request seriously, whether it was astrologically motivated or not, is of course somewhat doubtful, but the indication is in the chart.

The optimal time for the operation calculated on the basis of the Moon and Mars positions is fifteen weeks after the question, and this also has the advantage of Mars no longer being near the dangerous fixed stars around 25 Taurus (Capulus and Algol). The fifteen-degree distance the Moon has to cover before reaching the ascendant will stand for weeks; this is the only time unit which makes sense in this context. The operation was carried out in the calculated week and was totally successful without any complications.

Later on this client asked again about the operation on the right eye. In this chart the Sun is the relevant significator, which is always the right eye in males. The Sun is at 17 Taurus on the descendant and this looks threatening. From about 22 Taurus the Sun will enter the region around the extremely malefic fixed star Algol. The operation has to be carried out before this happens, so within five weeks.

More urgent however is the fact that the Sun is setting which would make it much weaker: the light in the eyes is disappearing. To prevent this from happening the operation has to take place as soon as possible. Another indication for this is retrograde Jupiter right on the ascendant. Whatever this means, it is in a positive reception with Mars, the operation. Jupiter is the Great Benefic; it has term dignity and is accidentally strong on the ascendant. It has some power to support Mars and it would be a good idea to make use of this power. So we have to act as soon as possible and to keep Jupiter out of the harmful and laming twelfth house.

Mars, the operation itself, has a rather neutral position here, but it is not in negative reception with the eye. Despite the fact that Mars is the ruler of the first house, we can take it as the operation. The central point of the question is the way the operation affects the eye so we can look at the relation between Mars and the Sun which symbolizes the eye. The operation took place as soon as possible, with good results but there was

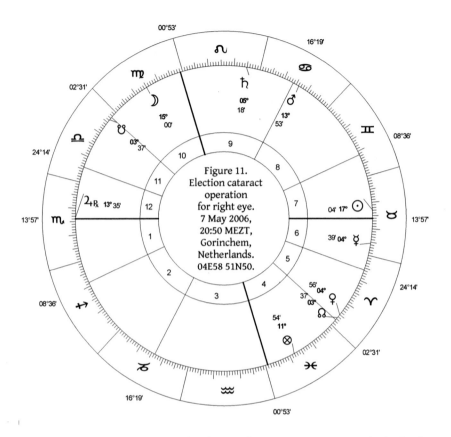

Figure 11.
Election cataract
operation
for right eye.
7 May 2006,
20:50 MEZT,
Gorinchem,
Netherlands.
04E58 51N50.

a small complication. Sun on the descendant in opposition with the body (ascendant) is less favourable than in conjunction with the ascendant. The client was able to choose the time of the operation with some detail because it was in a private clinic.

In this case we can also avail ourselves of the healing power of stones in preparing the eye for the operation and in strengthening the eye as after-care. A suitable stone which refers to vision in the Hildegard system is the gold topaz (a stone with a Sun signature). It should be worn on the skin, but can also be used to make gold topaz wine. We lay the stone in wine for a few days to infuse the wine with the stone's healing power. The eye-lid is moistened with the wine a few times a day until the complaints have disappeared or the period of recovery is over, (the wine has to be made again and again). Other stones besides gold topaz which can heal short-sightedness and weakening eyesight are hyacinth (zircon), beryl and agate.

12

Prevention

The constitution
This last chapter is about natal astrology as this is where we can give preventative advice. Medical astrology is practical and a medical horary enables us to make a diagnosis, as described in Chapter 4. However by assessing the temperament and analysing the role of the sixth house of disease in the natal chart, the weak points in the constitution can be found and preventive dietary and life-style advice can be given. Progressions and solar return charts also show when these weak points will come to the fore.

The first part of the medical analysis of the natal chart involves assessing the temperament. The temperament shows the humoral combination of the individual, it is the basic material and very important; it is the foundation for further delineation of the chart. A dominantly choleric person differs considerably from a dominantly phlegmatic person. Choleric individuals will be active and combative whereas phlegmatics will be soft and emotional and avoid conflicts and too much activity. This is also the foundation for traditional psychology which can give a clear psychological description of individual behaviour.

Also, in a medical sense, the temperament is the starting-point. The more balanced the humors in the natal chart, the stronger the constitution. Someone with a chart in which the four humors are evenly distributed will not be as vulnerable to disease as an individual with a yellow choler excess. This person will tend to develop fiery conditions. If we know this we can give preventive advice, for example a diet with more moistening and cooling foods, a lot of exercise and a blue or green precious stone to diminish the fiery tendencies.

In this way we can prevent the in-born humoral imbalance from developing into a real disease. It is important also to keep an eye on the secondary progressions of Sun, Moon, Asc, MC, (angles progressed by Nailbod in right ascension), Pars Fortunae and Lords 1 and 6. If these progressions aspect, for example, a position like Mars in Sagittarius in a temperament which is choleric, there is a chance that this person will have an illness which is caused by too much heat; the progressed aspect on Mars will introduce a lot of Fire into the body. When the progressed aspect becomes full, moistening and cooling foods should be eaten. If planets in the solar return also aspect this Mars position the danger of disease will become acute.

Furthermore we have to look at the position and dignity of Lord 6 and the influence of the planets in the sixth house. In the natal chart the sixth house does indicate disease, so this differs from the horary chart analysis. A natal chart is about the whole life and the houses refer to the specific aspects of life. Lord 6 and the planets in the sixth house have to be evaluated by their aspects and receptions especially with Lord 1 (the body) and the Lights Sun and Moon; these are the sources of the vital energy in the body.

We have to take into account the essential dignity of Lord 6 or planets in the sixth house. A planet with lots of essential dignity will not be too dangerous for the body. This also differs from the medical horary. In a natal chart, Jupiter in Pisces as the ruler of the sixth house will not cause many problems, whereas Saturn in detriment in Leo will soon lead to ill health.

The way Lord 6 and planets in the sixth house work out is assessed within the broader framework of the whole temperament, just like the other houses in the natal chart. In a balanced temperament Lord 6 will not cause problems as quickly as it would in a severely unbalanced temperament. If Lord 6 is Mars in Leo, this give the possibility of Fire diseases, but this danger increases considerably if the temperament is strongly choleric. The reverse can also be the case, because in a very phlegmatic temperament a fiery Lord 6 will lead to problems; it is like throwing a red-hot stone into a quiet cool pool.

Apart from the temperament and the sixth house there are two Arabic points which are of importance in the medical delineation of the natal chart: the Part of Illness where the misery of disease comes in, and the Part of Surgery/Treatment where we fight the disease. (This Part was used in the horary chart about the osteoporosis). If the Part of Illness is in narrow aspect with a planet or important point, it shows that disease will be an important theme in life. An aspect (orb less than two degrees) will bring disease more to the fore. As always we have to analyse this together with the temperament and the sixth house. The Part of Surgery/Treatment shows something about the power and nature of treatment and other medical interferences.

As the dispositor (sign ruler) of a Part represents it in the chart, we must also look at the dispositors. If there are no narrow aspects on the Parts themselves they will be less important, however. The formula for the Part of Illness in day charts is Asc + Mars - Saturn and for the Part of Surgery/Treatment Asc + Saturn – Mars. If the Sun is under the horizon (night chart), these formulae are reversed. The Part of Illness will then be Asc + Saturn - Mars and the Part of Surgery/Treatment Asc + Mars – Saturn.

Assessing the temperament

To assess the temperament we need to analyse five factors: the sign on the ascendant, the ruler of the first house, the Sun, the Moon, and the so-called Lord of the Geniture. The Lord of the Geniture is the planet with the most essential and accidental dignities in the chart. These five points are all separate factors of equal value which contribute to the overall temperament and can best be placed in columns in a table. In this way you will have five independent contributions to the temperament in terms of the humors, to give insight into the individual "basic material".

In assessing the temperament we have the following rules: the Sun contributes depending on the season, so when the Sun is in Aries, Taurus and Gemini it is sanguine; in Cancer, Leo and Virgo it is choleric; in Libra, Scorpio and Sagittarius it is melancholic; and in Capricorn, Aquarius and Pisces it is phlegmatic. Sanguine is hot and moist, choleric hot and dry, melancholic cold and dry and phlegmatic cold and moist. The Moon is assessed by phase: New Moon to first quarter is sanguine, from first quarter to Full Moon choleric, from Full Moon to last quarter melancholic and the last phase is phlegmatic.

The ascendant is assessed on the basis of the element of its sign, and Lord 1 and the Lord of the Geniture on the basis of their natures and their positions relative to the Sun. If we turn the natal chart to place the

Sun on the ascendant, any planet that appears above the horizon in the upper half of the chart is oriental; otherwise the planet is occidental. The meaning of oriental is rising before the Sun. An oriental planet will keep its own temperature, an occidental planet will take on the temperature of the sign in which it is placed. This is at least one of the versions of the traditional method.

Each factor is further qualified by narrow aspects (orb not much more than four degrees) and the sign in which it is placed. For planets in their roles as Lord 1 and the Lord of the Geniture we have the following natures: the Sun is always warm and dry, the Moon always moist and cold. Oriental positions: Mercury warm (moist or dry is determined by the sign background), Venus warm and moist, Mars warm and dry, Jupiter warm and moist, Saturn cold and moist. Occidental positions: Mercury dry, Venus moist, Mars dry, Jupiter moist, Saturn dry. The sign background will show whether the planet is cold or warm.

This is one of the methods traditionally used to assess temperament but there are some weak points. The fact that oriental Venus would be warm and moist instead of cold and moist and oriental Saturn cold and moist instead of cold and dry is rather dubious. Also the idea that an occidental planet would take on the heat or cold of its sign is debatable. There is no clarity about this. The only thing we can do is to compare several versions of the method in practice.

A version proposed by the Dutch classical astrologer George van Zanten is always to take the planets in their roles as Lord of the Geniture and Lord 1 according to their nature. So Saturn will always attribute black choler to the temperament irrespective of its position relative to the Sun. While in some charts this method gives a somewhat different temperament, it is a very logical idea and is worthwhile testing. The lack of clarity about the method is not such a problem in practice; we can use it for insight even if it is not 100% accurate. The following example shows how preventive advice is based on the analysis of the temperament and the sixth house. Firstly, we assess the temperament (natal chart "yellow choler" in figure 15).

Sun in Virgo, a summer sign, hot and dry: HD
Moon between first quarter and Full Moon (the "summer phase")
   hot and dry: HD
Ascendant Leo, a Fire sign, hot and dry: HD

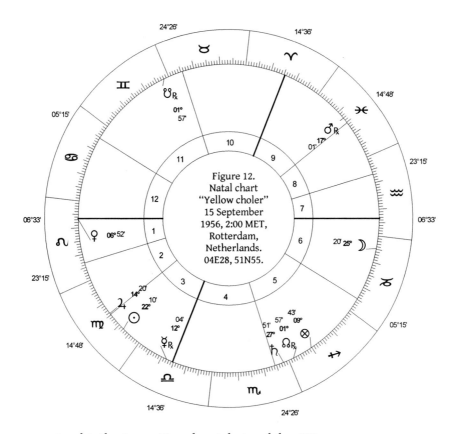

Figure 12.
Natal chart
"Yellow choler"
15 September
1956, 2:00 MET,
Rotterdam,
Netherlands.
04E28, 51N55.

Lord 1, the Sun, a Fire planet, hot and dry: HD

Lord of the Geniture (the planet with the most essential and accidental dignity) is occidental Mercury: dry in Libra a hot/moist sign so this adds heat: HD. (In the Van Zanten-method this would give black choler; the other factors would not change).

All the five factors are choleric, a very unbalanced temperament, which greatly increases the chances of falling ill. Preventively we would have to add extra moist and cold foods to the diet, certainly in the yellow choler phase with its dominating Fire tendency which starts with puberty. This client did indeed develop a chronic disease around the age of twenty.

Yellow choler excess

After many years of trying all kind of non-alternative and alternative treatments, this client came to my practice with a medical horary question. The horary chart indicated that the cause of the problem was black choler and the measures against the excess of melancholy did have more effect than the client had experienced for a long time. The fact that the problem is caused by excess melancholy can be seen in the natal chart in the sixth house.

The sixth house ruler is Saturn, a cold and dry planet in a cold and moist sign. The planet in the sixth house is the Moon in Capricorn, an extremely cold and dry sign. The Moon and Saturn both have little dignity, the Moon being in detriment and Saturn only in term. This makes the Moon especially extremely harmful. Lord 1, the Sun, is in narrow aspect with the Moon and with Saturn and this connects the body with a lot of cold and dryness. There is clearly the threat of cold and dry, melancholic diseases.

However, this has to be assessed in the broader framework of the overall temperament which is extremely choleric. This intensive heat will burn the body up and what we are left with after the fire is black choler; the body has been burnt up from inside. If yellow choler is not tempered and burns on unhindered for a long time, we end up with a melancholic excess. The strongly melancholic factor connected with the sixth house of diseases make this potential danger acute; the illness tendencies are evaluated on the basis of the temperament and the sixth house together.

In this case a preventive astromedical consultation could have been of great value. The temperament is so unbalanced and the sixth house so threatening that we can clearly see that there is a great danger of the development of chronic diseases even at an early age. If measures against yellow and black choler had been taken in youth as described in Part 3 of this book, such a disease would probably not have developed. It is striking that the first diseases began to manifest early in the choleric phase of puberty and adolescence. Yellow choler dominates this phase of life; it will increase the amount of yellow choler which is present in the temperament and will disturb the balance in the body definitively.

The asthmatic writer
Another interesting chart as regards disease and prevention is that of the French writer Marcel Proust. In his semi-autobiographical work we meet the author as an imaginative and sharply observing individual

who was brought up in an overly protective atmosphere. He was very sickly and at an early age suffered from severe lung problems; asthmatic complaints that would continue all his life. His chart clearly shows where the problem originated and also what could have been done to prevent it. The first step is again assessment of the temperament.

Sun is in Cancer, a summer sign which gives heat and dryness:
    HD, choleric.
Moon between last quarter and new Moon, moisture and cold:
    CM, phlegmatic.
Aries on the ascendant, Fire sign, gives heat and dryness: HD,
    choleric.
Mars, Lord 1 rising after the Sun, occidental heat and dryness:
    HD, choleric.

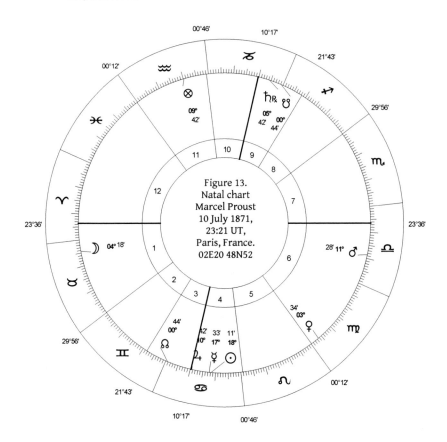

Figure 13. Natal chart Marcel Proust 10 July 1871, 23:21 UT, Paris, France. 02E20 48N52

Lord of the Geniture Jupiter, oriental, heat and moisture: HM, sanguine. (The Van Zanten method gives the same temperament here).

Choleric again but not as unbalanced as the last case. The assessment of the temperament can be refined further on the basis of aspects and sign placement. These refinements do not change the nature of the humor but they can temper or emphasise certain facets. Sometimes this can help in determining which humor dominates; orbs should be kept small, a maximum of four or five degrees.

The Sun in cold and moist Cancer will be less hot and dry because of this sign placement, it is not HD, but H-D-. Also the conjunction with cold and dry Mercury will bring some extra melancholy, H-D- becomes H- - D. There are no further narrow aspects so the contribution of the Sun to the temperament is less warm but remains dry.

The Moon is CM, in a cold and dry sign (Taurus) so it will be colder but less moist: C+ M-. The trine with Venus gives more moisture and cold: C++ M and the trine with Saturn more cold and dryness C+++ M-. So the Moon is very cold but less moist.

Ascendant is hot and dry, conjunct the antiscion of cold and moist Venus, so H-D-.

Lord 1 is hot and dry in a hot and moist sign; this makes it warmer but less dry: H+ D-, the square with hot and moist Jupiter adds some heat and moisture: H++D--.

Lord of the Geniture Jupiter is warm and moist in a cold and moist sign, so H- M+, the square with Mars gives heat and dryness: HM.

This refinement shows that there is less dryness while the cold of the Moon is strong. All in all it makes the hot and dry temperament somewhat more balanced, also because the dryness is tempered. Psychologically Proust is an active combative choleric with some soft spots; the phlegmatic sensitive Moon and the social, merrily dynamic Jupiter. Because the sanguine Jupiter is placed on cusp 4, the sanguine nature will show itself more at home than in public.

Medically his temperament is unbalanced, which points to the risk of disease if other relevant significators confirm this tendency. We have to look at the sixth house and its ruler; Venus in Virgo is close to the 6th house cusp, a cold and moist planet in a cold and dry sign, in its fall, which makes it harmful. Venus is on the ascendant by antiscion (planet positions mirrored in the Cancer/Capricorn axis); the illness planet affects the body directly. Mercury/Lord 6 is in cold and moist Cancer, the sign of the lungs and in the fourth house, of the lungs. In the same sign and house there are two more planets in Cancer, which bring more slime into the lungs.

The Moon/Lord 4 narrowly aspects this nasty Venus in the sixth house which connects cold diseases with the lungs. Lord 1, the body, is in detriment in the sixth house and the planets in Cancer receive this weak Lord 1 into fall and so harm the body. There are many indicators for severe illness, but the final touch is the Part of Illness which conjuncts Lord 6 in the fourth house and emphasises the illness theme.

The problem we read in this chart is too much phlegm in the lungs. The preventive treatment would have to be directed at reducing the amount of phlegm at the time of activation of these positions. Although Proust is dominantly choleric by temperament, his illness concentrates around phlegmatic excess. This may sound strange but people with excess yellow choler are also extra sensitive to phlegm diseases. Basic prevention however would have to be oriented on creating more balance in the excessively hot and dry temperament. Another good preventive measure would be the wearing of an apophyllite, a cooling precious stone which works against too much phlegm.

Conclusion: What is classical astrology?

This book has been explicitly about classical astrology and in some readers this will trigger the question, 'What is this?' Classical astrology is astrology as it existed for more than twenty centuries in the west, with its last heyday in the seventeenth century, mainly in England. After that, science and the "Enlightenment" pushed aside the traditional world view. Astrology appeared again on the scene in the late nineteenth century, mainly through the work of a group of English theosophists including Alan Leo.

Although these theosophists knew the traditional books to some extent, they changed almost everything according to their own tastes and prejudices and what they created hardly resembled the astrology that had gone before. This radical theosophical reconstruction has developed into what we call modern astrology and in the twentieth century many new age and psychological ideas were added to it. Classical astrology bases itself on the tradition as it existed before this reconstruction and it only uses as its sources texts and practices from the seventeenth century and earlier periods.

This immediately points to the danger that classical astrology might develop into an academic discipline of dry text researchers who fight each other with their Greek and Arabic citations. The real tradition is a living tradition, classical methods as they were described in the old texts are the starting-point indeed, but they have to be evaluated critically, they have to be tested in practice and if necessary adapted so that they will work. Traditional authors were human beings like us; they were not prophets or gods who wrote down the "Absolute Truth". Books do give us a foundation to stand on, but practice and logic are also necessary for an effective classical astrology. This is inevitable because the old texts are incomplete and they contradict each other on many points. This approach seems to lead to good results – as you will be able to check for yourself by using this book.

Appendix A

Stars Associated with Blindness

A considerable number of fixed stars carry the meaning of blindness, especially star nebulas because of their nebulous signature. Blindness can be taken literally or metaphorically when analysing charts, but in most cases the metaphorical meaning will be the most relevant. However, in a medical context the literal meaning does often play a role, especially in questions about eye operations. We have to check carefully in these questions or in elections if blindness stars come into play. A narrow orb applies, one degree for most stars, although we can use an orb of two or three degrees for the more powerful first-magnitude stars and especially for the influential stars mentioned in Part 1 of this book. The following list gives the positions of the stars associated with blindness:

Vertex (nebula)	27 Aries
Capulus (cluster)	24 Taurus
Alcyone/Pleiades (cluster)	29 Taurus/0 Gemini
Hyads (cluster)	6 Gemini
Ensis (nebula)	23 Gemini
Praesepe with S.Asellus (cluster)	7 Leo
Copula (nebula)	25 Virgo
Foramen (nebula)	22 Libra
Aculeus (cluster)	25 Sagittarius
Acumen (cluster)	28 Sagittarius
Spiculum (nebula)	0 Capricorn
Facies (cluster)	8 Capricorn
Manubrium (cluster)	14 Capricorn

Fixed stars are not really fixed, they move at a slow pace of about 1 degree every 72 years, so we have to correct the positions for this time factor. The positions mentioned above are those for the year of the writing of this book (2007). The stars which carry the meaning of blindness are all nebulas or nebulous star clusters, groups of stars heaped together embedded in a cloud of dust. If we look at the Pleiades we can see this quite clearly, even without binoculars. The signature of nebulousness refers to the decreased eye sight these stars tend to cause.

The most powerful blindness star is Alcyone and it will have a powerful influence on the interpretation of the chart, even if the question is not explicitly about the eyes or related matters. The other stars can be discarded; only if the client asks explicitly about the eye-sight or seeing in a literal or metaphorical sense should they be taken into account.

Appendix B

How to Spot Body Types

The temperament which can be assessed using the method described in Part 4 of this book can be seen not only in the behaviour but also in the appearance and the physical build. The strongly mixed types are not as easy to spot as those who are more unbalanced. The influence of the sign on the ascendant on the appearance is a bit stronger than that of the other factors in the temperament. Often you can recognize some typical characteristics of the ascending sign in the face. With some experience it is possible to quickly recognise the dominant inbuilt humor and behaviour.

This is very useful, because you then know the best way to approach such a person. It is not smart to be too direct to a phlegmatic, unless you want to silence him. From a person with a dry skin, piercing eyes and a loud voice and laugh, you can expect sharp comments so it is not a good idea to draw him out too much, unless you are deliberately trying to provoke him of course.

General principles can be helpful in spotting the dominant humor. The simple questions to start with are: how long and how corpulent is the body? Height gives an indication of heat or cold, heat shortens, cold makes longer. The amount of fat says something about the moisture content as moisture expands, dryness keeps to a straight line; moisture connects and crosses borders. This is the reason some people can eat anything and still not put on weight, whereas others have to closely watch what they eat. These two simple horizontal and vertical dimensions will clarify a lot about the temperamental make-up. Of course we have to take into account the age as older bodies are drier than younger bodies.

The extreme melancholics (the dominant humor in astrological circles) can be spotted quite easily. They tend to be slim, sometimes even skinny; often they are long, behave laconically and tend to have a dry wit. It is also important to take into account the family background. A dry and cold type from a family with many small people will not be as long as a melancholic from a tall family. Moreover, a planet in narrow aspect with the ascendant strongly affects the appearance. This will sometimes make the impression confusing.

Cholerics: dry, reddish skin, loud voice and laugh, sharp eyes, big hands, not too long, not slim but not corpulent, good strong muscles, sporty, combative, cat-like.

Phlegmatics: moist pale skin, the notorious weak hand-shake, flabby, not long but big (but not always, they may be small), formless, soft voice, moist friendly eyes, small hands, easy to intimidate, soft, wants to connect emotionally, cute, look younger than they are.

Sanguines: moist skin not pale, playful eyes, small hands, friendly, enthusiastic, more flesh but not flabby, not long, active, social, talks a lot.

Melancholics: drier skin, but not reddish (even pale), slim or skinny, often very tall (but not always), laconic behaviour, the huge "beanpole", excessive dark hair, long hands with slender fingers, sad eyes, does not talk much, wary, dry wit.

Naturally, every type may put on weight and even the places on the body where the fat appears is characteristic of the body type. Phlegmatics however are the most sensitive to weight-gain because of their slow metabolism. Because the temperament describes the basic building materials out of which an individual is formed, the temperament in general relates to the whole body.

Epilogue

I have said what I wanted to say, so now I will be silent. My famous forerunner Nicholas Culpeper will close my book with the words that are found on the first page of his *Astrological Judgement of Diseases* from the *Decumbiture of The Sick:*

> "To you all, and to you especially that heard these lectures do I dedicate them and present them to you not to look upon only (for then I had as good have sent you a picture, and as much it would have pleased your eye). Man was made not onely for speculation, but also for practise; speculation brings only pleasure to a man's self, it's practise which benefits others And I hope I need not tell you that man was not born for himself alone."

Glossary

Accidental dignity	Power of manifestation of a planet in the world.
Affliction	Harm done to a planet or point which leads to decreased effectiveness.
Antiscion	Mirrored planet position around Capricorn/ Cancer axis.
Aspect	Connection between planets through their angular distance (for example 90 or 180 degrees).
Ayurveda	Traditional form of healing in India.
Benefic	Planet with positive effect because of its nature or dignity.
Black choler	Earth, cold and dry.
Blood	Air, moist and warm.
Cazimi	Planet position within 17.30 minutes of arc from the exact centre of the Sun; powerful.
Collection of light	A third planet connecting two others because it is aspected by them.
Combust	Planet position within 8.30 degrees from the Sun; weakening.
Cusp	Starting point of a house.
Debility	Negative dignity, weakening.
Decanate (face)	Zone of ten degrees in a sign.
Decumbiture	Chart for the moment of "falling ill".
Detriment	Strong essential debility; harmful.
Dispositor	The rulers of the sign a planet is placed in.
Dosha	A humor in Ayurveda.
Electional astrology	Choosing the most favourable chart for commencing something.
Essential dignity	Degree of quality of a planet.
Exaltation	A powerful essential dignity.

Face	See decanate.
Fall	Strong essential debility.
Horary astrology	Astrology dealing with question charts.
House ruler	Planet ruling the sign on the house cusp.
Humor	Body fluid, element in the body.
Joy	Accidental dignity because of house position.
Lunation	Full Moon or New Moon.
Malefic	Planet with negative effect because of its nature or debility.
Mundane astrology	The astrology of world affairs and politics.
Mutual reception	Planets in each other's essential dignities.
Natal astrology	The delineation of birth charts.
Orb	Number of degrees within which a planet has an effect.
Pars	Arabian point, part or lot.
Partile	Aspect made by planets in the same degree of their respective signs.
Peregrine	Without essential dignity; not debilitated.
Phlegm	Slime, Water, cold and moist.
Prohibition	A planet preventing an aspect.
Purging	Removing a harmful humor from the body.
Reception	Effect of one planet on a second planet by placement in the second planet's dignity.
Retrogradation	A planet moving backward; accidental debility.
Sign ruler	The big boss of a sign.
Solar return chart	Predictive chart for a year in natal astrology based on the birthday.
Stationary	Planet reversing its direction; weak.
Term	A weak essential dignity; gives a small amount of power.
Term ruler	Planet ruling the term a planet is placed in.
Translation of light	A third planet connecting two others by aspecting them.
Triplicity	Element.
Triplicity ruler	The planet ruling the element by day or by night.
Unani	Traditional humoral form of medicine in South Asia.

Under the Sun's beams	Position between 8.30 and 17.30 degrees from the Sun; weakening.
Vedic astrology	Traditional astrology of India.
Via combusta	The "burnt road"; weak place for the Moon (15 Libra to 15 Scorpio).
Void of course	A planet no longer making any aspect in the sign in which it is placed.
Yellow choler	Fire, hot and dry.

Bibliography

Avicenna, *The Canon of Medicine*, KAZI Publications, Chicago, USA, 1999.

Hildegard von Bingen, *Das Buch von den Steinen*, originally 12th century, Otto Müller Verlag, Salzburg, Austria, 1997.

Al Biruni, *Elements of the Art of Astrology*, originally 1029, facsimile edition, Ascella, London, England, 2001.

Joseph Blagrave, *Astrological Practise of Physic*, originally 1671, facsimile edition, Ascella, London, England, 2001.

Hakim G.M. Chisti, *The Traditional Healer's Handbook*, Healing Arts Press, Rochester, Vermont, USA, 1988.

Nicholas Culpeper, *Complete Herbal*, originally 1653, Foulsham & Co. Ltd, Berks, England.

_____ *Astrological Judgement of Diseases from the Decumbiture of the Sick*, originally 1655, facsimile edition, Ascella, London, England, 2001.

Firmicus Maternus, *Matheseos Libri 8*, originally fourth century, Ascella, London, England, 1995.

John Frawley, *The Real Astrology*, Apprentice Books, London, England, 2000.

_____ *The Real Astrology Applied*, Apprentice Books, London, England, 2002.

_____ *The Horary Textbook*, Apprentice Books, London, England, 2005.

Friedemann Garvelmann, *Pflanzenheilkunde in der Humoralpathologie*, Pflaum Verlag, München, Germany, 2000.

Michael Gienger, *Steinheilkunde*, Neue Erde, Saarbrücken, Germany, 1995.

Michael Gienger, *Lexikon der Heilsteine*, Neue Erde, Saarbrücken, Germany, 1996.

Peter Hochmeier, *Der Weg des Sonnenfunkens*, Bacopa Verlag, Schiedlberg, Austria, 1996.

Abraham Ibn Ezra, *The Beginning of Wisdom*, originally 12th century, facsimile John Hopkins Press/Oxford University Press 1939, Ascella, London, England.

Harish Johari, *The Healing Power of Gemstones in Tantra, Ayurveda and Astrology*, Destiny Books, Rochester, Vermont, USA, 1988.

William Lilly, *Christian Astrology Books 1, 2 & 3*, originally 1647, Ascella, London, England, 2001.

Richard Saunders, *The Astrological Judgement and Practise of Physick*, originally 1677, Ascella, London, England, 2001.

Djalaloed-dien Abdoer-Rahman As-Soejoethi, *De Geneeskunde van de Profeet (Medicine of the Prophet)*, originally 15th century, Noer, Delft, The Netherlands, 2004.

Wighard Strehlow, *Die Psychotherapie der Hildegard von Bingen*, Heilen mit der Kraft der Seele, Lüchow Verlag, Stuttgart, Germany, 2004.

Wighard Strehlow, *Die Edelsteinheilkunde der Hildegard von Bingen*, Lüchow Verlag, Stuttgart, Germany, 2004.

Graem Tobyn, *Culpeper's Medicine*, Element Books, Shaftesbury, England, 1997.

Index

affliction, 50, 72
Air, 3, 9, 12, *see also* Chapters 1, 14
Air planet, 12, 21
Air signs, 32, 48
alchemy, 81
Alcyone, 36, 127
Aldebaran, 36
Algol, 35, 36
anatomy, 18-19
Antares, 36
antipathy, 59-61
antiscia, 55
Arabian parts
  of illness, 118-119
  of treatment/surgery, 106
arthritis, 42
aspects, 35
  on parts, 119
  with Lord, 6, 118
  with the Moon, 48
astrology
  classical, 125
  modern medical, 3
  Vedic, 92, 96
Ayurvedic medicine, 11, 25, 30
benefic, 34
besiegement, 35, 55
black choler, 10-11, *see also* Chapter 1
Blagrave, Joseph, 64
blindness, 36, 127
blood, 9-10, *see also* Chapter 1
blood-letting, 16, 80-81
body type, 129
cardinal sign, 51, 62
cataract, 113
cause of disease, 41, 45, 47
cazimi, 35
charts
  arthritis, 43
  election cataract operation left
    eye, 113
  election cataract operation right
    eye, 116

iliac passion, 57
multiple sclerosis, 49
osteoporosis, 47
psoriasis, 54
Proust, Marcel, natal chart, 123
sinusitis, 108
womb operation, 112
yellow choler, natal chart, 121
choleric, 5, *see also* Chapter 1
classical astrology, 18, 29, 84, 125
cold, 5, *see also* Chapter 1
conjunction
  with antiscia, 55
  with the Sun and the nodal axis, 35
constitution, 117
crystals, 45, 64, 85
Culpeper, Nicholas, 61-64
cusp, 44, 58
day chart, 32
debilitation, 34, 35
decanate, 32, 34
decumbiture, 39
detriment, 30-31
diagnosis, 3, 29, 38
diet, 45, 55, 56, 59, 66
digestion, 9, 87
dignity
  accidental, 34-35
  essential, 30-35
disposition, 106
dispositor, 37, 41, 45
dosha, 11
dry, 5, *see also* Chapter 1
Earth, 3, *see also* Chapters 1, 14
Earth planets, 38
Earth signs, 32, 43
election, 110-116
element, 3, *see also* Chapter 1
essence, 45, 82-83
ether, 12
exaltation, 30-31
face, 32-33
fall, 31

Fire, 3, 6, *see also* Chapters 1, 14
fixed signs, 52, 55, 77
fixed stars, 35, 36, 114, 115
foods, classification of, 66-67
Freud, Sigmund, 89
heat, 5, *see also* Chapter 1
herbs, 74-76
homoeopathy, 63, 81
hormonal glands, 24, 93
house
    anatomical, 18-19
    sixth, 38, 39, 117-118
humor, 4, *see also* Chapter 1
iliac passion, 57
infections, 16-17
joy, 35
Jupiter, 21
life style, 70, 85
Lilly, William, 39, 96
liver, 9-10
lord of the geniture, 119-120
Lucifer, 91
Mars, 20-21
melancholy, 10-11, *see also* Chapter 1
Mercury, 21-22
metals, 94-95
moist, 5, *see also* Chapter 1
Moon, 22, 31, 38, 47
multiple sclerosis, 48
mundane astrology, 14
mutable signs, 51, 53
natal chart, 29, 39, 118
night chart, 32
occidental, 120
operations, questions about, 105
opposition
    of signs, 63
    with the Sun, 3
orb
    antiscion, 119
    aspect, 120
    cazimi, 35
    combustion, 35
    cusp, 111
    fixed stars, 127
organs, 20-22
oriental, 120

outer planets, 24
parathyroid gland, 106
peregrine, 34
phlegm, 7-8, *see also* Chapter 1
Placidus, 80
planetary hours, 79
planets, 16, 18-22
Pluto, 114
precious stones, 84, 91, *see also*
    Chapter 9
prevention, 117, *see also* Chapter 12
prognosis, 36, 50, 53
progression, 29, 117
Proust, Marcel, 122-123
psoriasis, 7, 53
psychology, traditional, 72, 85, 117
purge, to, 76, 91
quintessence, 12
receptions, 37
Regulus, 35
retrograde, 36, 48, 50-51, 114
ruler, 18, 20
sanguine, 9-10, *see also* Chapter 1
Saturn, 20
sauna, 67, 71, 85
Saunders, Richard, 29, 41-43, 92
sextile, 58, 112
signature, 61-62, 86, 92
sin, 85
sinusitis, 7, 96
slime, 4, 7-8, *see also* Chapter 1
solar return chart, 117
soul therapy, 84, 89
spagyric, 75, 81-83
speed, 50
Spica, 35, 36, 11, 112
square, 40, 51, 52
stationary, 36
Sun, 21, 32, 34, 35, 38
surgery, 105, 106, 113
sympathy, 60-61
symptom, 13-14
temperament, 117, *see also* Chapter 12
term, 32-34
timing, 52, 11
tincture, 45, 63, 81-82
traditional Chinese medicine, 11, 30

treatment plan, 45, 56
treatments, questions about, 105
trine, 124
triplicity, 32
turning the chart, 107
Unani, 30, 76-77
under the Sun's beams, 35
Venus, 20, 21
vertebrae, 85
via combusta, 35
Vindemiatrix, 36
virtue, 85
von Bingen, Hildegard, 84, 91
Water, 3, 7-8, *see also* Chapter 1, 14
yellow choler, 5, *see also* Chapter 1

Other Books by The Wessex Astrologer

The Essentials of Vedic Astrology
Lunar Nodes - Crisis and Redemption
Personal Panchanga and the Five
Sources of Light
Komilla Sutton

Astrolocality Astrology
From Here to There
Martin Davis

The Consultation Chart
Introduction to Medical Astrology
Wanda Sellar

The Betz Placidus Table of Houses
Martha Betz

Astrology and Meditation
Greg Bogart

Patterns of the Past
Karmic Connections
Good Vibrations
Soulmates and why to avoid them
Judy Hall

The Book of World Horoscopes
Nicholas Campion

The Moment of Astrology
Geoffrey Cornelius

Life After Grief - An Astrological
Guide to Dealing with Loss
AstroGraphology - The Hidden link
between your Horoscope and your
Handwriting
Darrelyn Gunzburg

The Houses: Temples of the Sky
Deborah Houlding

Temperament: Astrology's
Forgotten Key
Dorian Geiseler Greenbaum

Astrology, A Place in Chaos
Star and Planet Combinations
Bernadette Brady

Astrology and the Causes of War
Jamie Macphail

Flirting with the Zodiac
Kim Farnell

The Gods of Change
Howard Sasportas

Astrological Roots:
The Hellenistic Legacy
Joseph Crane

The Art of Forecasting
using Solar Returns
Anthony Louis

Horary Astrology Re-Examined
Barbara Dunn

Living Lilith - Four Dimensions of the
Cosmic Feminine
M. Kelley Hunter

Your Horoscope in Your Hands
Lorna Green

Primary Directions
Martin Gansten

www.wessexastrologer.com

LaVergne, TN USA
18 April 2010
179658LV00002B/6/P

9 781902 405407